The Encyclopedia *of* Ayurvedic Massage

Other books by John Douillard:

Perfect Health for Kids:
Ten Ayurvedic Health Secrets Every Parent Must Know

The 3-Season Diet:
Eat the Way Nature Intended
to Lose Weight, Beat Cravings, and Get Fit

Body, Mind, and Sport:
The Mind-Body Guide to Lifelong Fitness
and Your Personal Best

The Encyclopedia of Ayurvedic Massage

DR. JOHN DOUILLARD

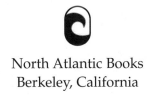

North Atlantic Books
Berkeley, California

Published by North Atlantic Books

North Atlantic Books   Cover and book design by Suzanne Albertson
P.O. Box 12327   Cover photo © Picture Quest
Berkeley, California 94712   Printed in the United States of America

Although anyone may find the suggestions in this book useful and beneficial, they are not intended as a diagnosis, prescription, recommended treatment or cure for any specific problem, whether medical, emotional, psychological, social or spiritual. This book was written for educational purposes only and not designed to replace therapy or consultation with a qualified professional.

The Encyclopedia of Ayurvedic Massage is sponsored by the Society for the Study of Native Arts and Sciences, a nonprofit educational corporation whose goals are to develop an educational and crosscultural perspective linking various scientific, social, and artistic fields; to nurture a holistic view of arts, sciences, humanities, and healing; and to publish and distribute literature on the relationship of mind, body, and nature.

North Atlantic Books' publications are available through most bookstores. For further information, call 800–733–3000 or visit our website at www.northatlanticbooks.com.

ISBN 13: 978-1-55643-493-8

Library of Congress Cataloging-in-Publication Data

Douillard, John.
    The encyclopedia of ayurvedic massage / by John Douillard.
        p.   cm.
        ISBN 1-55643-493-6 (pbk.)
    1. Massage—Encyclopedias. 2. Medicine, Ayurvedic—Encyclopedias.
    DNLM: 1. Massage—methods—Encyclopedias—English. 2. Medicine,
    Ayurvedic—Encyclopedias—English. WB 13 D737e 2004] I. Title.
RA780.5.D68 2004
615.8'22–dc22   2004004873

        3 4 5 6 7 8 9 10 11 12 13 14 DATA 14 13 12 11 10 09 08

TABLE OF CONTENTS

PART IV
Ayurvedic Therapies That Follow Massage

ACKNOWLEDGMENTS

In the eighteen years it has taken to write this book there are many to thank. First are all the Ayurvedic therapists I have worked with over the years who have put their heart and soul to every stroke year after year.

There are a few people I would like to thank whose efforts made this book a reality. Without them this book could still be years away.

Samara Frame for overseeing this entire project, orchestrating the layout, selecting the photos, merging photos with text, and for modeling.

Kate Fotopoulos for being the editor second to none. To edit this book Kate became an expert in the field of Ayurvedic massage. Her attention to perfected detail has made this book into the encyclopedia that it is.

Cathy Poole, who started practicing Ayurvedic massage in 1984, has brought twenty years of experience into the creation of this book. Cathy made certain that the incredible treatment experience we offer at LifeSpa was translated precisely into this work.

Thank you to Matt Safarik for his photo-shoot modeling.

Thank you to everyone at North Atlantic Books, especially Brooke Warner for her patience and personal tender loving care that was needed to make this book happen.

And last but by no means least, thank you to my family for motivating me to continue to write these books.

FOREWORD

In the West we are just beginning to appreciate the hidden pearls of wisdom sewn in the 5,000-year-old fabric of Ayurvedic medicine. To understand the difference between Eastern and Western mindsets, consider the fact that Ayurvedic massage practices, for example, are as much a part of daily life in India as is shampooing your hair in the United States. There are millions of elders in India who have had a massage or have massaged themselves since the day they were born. Imagine being eighty years old and having had a massage every day of your life—that comes to nearly 30,000 massages! This is commonplace in India.

Not only have these practices been time tested and proven throughout the ages, they were also developed based on principles that have only recently come into vogue in the West. Thousands of years ago the entire system of health care called Ayurveda evolved around the premise that mind, body, and spirit were one. Rather than thinking of them separately as we do in the West, Ayurveda has been treating them holistically, and Ayurvedic massage is just one element of the fabric that directly addresses the inseparable nature of mind, body, and spirit.

While I will elucidate the many pathways and mechanisms through which Ayurvedic massage attains these results, remember that Ayurveda has been practiced for thousands of years as one fabric—not three. As a result, experiencing the Ayurvedic massage techniques produces an integration of mind, body, and spirit unknown to most Westerners. I have been administering these treatments since 1986 and hear patients say every day that they have never felt so calm, gone so deep, been so still, or sensed such rejuvenation as when they finished an Ayurvedic massage.

This is the first time, to my knowledge, that these extremely detailed and coveted Ayurvedic massage descriptions have been published in such explicit detail. This encyclopedia is designed for massage or spa therapists and interested health care practitioners to instruct them in (not merely introduce them to) the world of Ayurvedic treatments. While each therapy is described step by step, with accompanying photographs, the information in this volume can never take the place of direct, hands-on, supervised instruction. At LifeSpa, we use this encyclopedia as our training manual for certifying practitioners in Ayurvedic massage.

I feel very honored to be able to present this therapeutic system in its fullness to the reader and have done so in the hopes of protecting the integrity of this very precious knowledge. These techniques were passed down from father to son for thousands of years, never leaving the trust of the family or tribe. I have been fortunate to have been privy to this knowledge for the past eighteen years. While Ayurveda is becoming more popular in the West, particularly in the spa and massage industries, I feel it is important that practitioners in these fields have an authentic body of knowledge to work from. These treatments as I describe them have a precise effect that will or will not be realized based on the intention and consciousness with which the therapies are offered. To insure that these therapies last another 5,000 years it is important that we in the West offer the treatments in the name of Ayurveda in the authentic nature in which they were passed on to us. Please use these Ayurvedic massage therapies with the gratitude and respect that a 5,000-year-old tradition deserves. It is that tradition that has made this encyclopedia possible.

—John Douillard
Boulder, Colorado
February 2004

HOW TO USE THIS BOOK

*T*he *Encyclopedia of Ayurvedic Massage* is not meant to take the place of hands-on instruction from an experienced Ayurvedic therapist, which has been the traditional means of transmitting this knowledge for thousands of years.

To derive the maximum benefit from this book, please take the time to read the introductory chapters to familiarize yourself with the history of Ayurvedic massage and the purpose of these therapeutic techniques. Pay special attention to Chapter 4, which discusses the different body types and the modifications each requires when performing the therapies.

Chapter 5 defines each stroke in detail and has illustrations showing hand positions and directions for the strokes. The chapters that follow have mostly small, thumbnail photographs, which serve to jog your memory during treatments. Chapters 6–16 outline the sequence of strokes using their names only and refer you back to the pages in Chapter 5 where those strokes were previously defined.

PART I

The Anatomy of Ayurvedic Massage

In Ayurvedic medicine, the role of massage involves much more than relieving stress, relaxing tight muscles, and reducing physical pain. Once balance in the physical body is restored, channels of circulation called *srotas* help to balance the three *doshas—Vata, Pitta,* and *Kapha.* At this point Ayurvedic massage begins to move the ten *vayus* or *pranas* that carry life force to both the physical and energetic bodies. Once the vayu function is optimal, the *nadi* system is activated. There are 72,000 nadis in the body that carry subtle energy. Specifically they carry consciousness to the *chakra* system and into the brain centers, where body, mind, and spirit are purified. The goal of this process is full human potential, whereby consciousness is lively in each and every cell. The subtle-body system and the physical body begin to function as one, resulting in perfect physical, mental, and spiritual health.

Chapter One

Introduction to Ayurvedic Medicine

It is clearly unique in this day and age to find a system of medicine that is thousands of years old and still one of the largest on the planet today. Ayurvedic medicine, although in its infancy here in America, has over 300,000 Indian doctors in the All Indian Ayurvedic Congress, making it the largest medical organization in the world. While the exact time and date of Ayurveda's arrival in India is unclear, most Western scholars agree that its onset was somewhere between 2500 and 600 B.C. Eastern scholars disagree and date Ayurvedic roots back as far as 4500 B.C. The *Rig Veda,* which may be the oldest repository of human knowledge in the world today, recorded an astrological phenomenon that date-maps these writings to earlier than 4,000 B.C.[1] While all such dating is somewhat unreliable, it is clear that Ayurveda is thousands of years old and that it had a developmental impact on the medicinal systems of Greece, Indonesia, China, and Persia.

Throughout the *Rig Veda,* Ayurvedic herbs are mentioned and praised for their ability both to cure and to prevent disease. Ayurvedic massage has its roots in *Siddha* medicine, a system of medicine that was brought to the south of India by the great *siddhar* or sage Agastya. It is said that Siddha medicine is the oldest system of medicine in the world, with siddhars claiming it to be 8,000 years old. It has two branches: Siddha medicine and Siddha massage. It is the latter branch of knowledge, written down on palm leaves and passed from master to disciple, that holds the roots to the Ayurvedic massage techniques and practices I will present in this manual. It was in the South under the auspices of Agastya and the eighteen great siddhars that the techniques of detoxification processes called *panchakarma* and *kya kalpa* were developed.

Over time, the two systems of medicines, Siddha and Ayurveda, overlapped, with Ayurveda predominantly in the North and Siddha in the South. Many of the massage treatments that originated as a part of Siddha medicine are practiced and taught today in both systems. This book reflects the current teachings of Ayurvedic medicine with great respect and gratitude for the wisdom of Siddha medicine from which much of today's Ayurvedic massage came.

Ayurveda

Ayurveda is a Sanskrit word derived from the roots *ayus* (life) and *veda* (knowledge). Knowledge arranged systematically with logic becomes science, and over time, Ayurveda became the science of life. It has its roots in ancient Vedic literature such as the *Rig Veda* and encompasses the entirety of human life—body, mind, and spirit.

The originator of the Ayurvedic system is *Brahma* (the Creator according to Vedic tradition) who passed it on to the *Aswini Kumars* (physicians of the Gods) who imparted the knowledge to the *Rishis* (seers by cognition) who in turn began teaching it to subsequent generations via an oral tradition, passing the knowledge from father to son. The amount of time from first cognition to first textbook is unknown.

At the turn of the first millennium B.C., two major Ayurvedic treatises were written. The first and still most important is called *Charaka Samhita*, which is a work primarily for physicians who are taught to diagnose and treat the body, mind, and spirit of the individual. The second major writing in Ayurveda is called *Sushrut Samhita,* which was the world's first recorded and comprehensive surgical text.

Sushrut also described the ancient *marmas* or vital points, which are believed to be the precursors to what is now practiced as acupuncture.[2] In the South, where it was first introduced, marma therapy played an important part in Siddha and Ayurvedic medicine. In the North, marma points were considered too delicate and powerful to treat, so marma therapy was assiduously avoided.

I was fortunate to receive my Ayurvedic training in a variety of locations across India. In the North I studied in New Delhi and Benares, in central India in Hydrabad, and in the South in Kerala. I was gifted with a broad view of therapeutic practices that were often in conflict with each other.

The cultures in northern and southern India are as different as the climates, and arguments still arise over disparities in therapeutic philosophies. When I co-directed Deepak Chopra's Ayurvedic center from 1986 to 1994, I revived a very successful marma therapy program that was in line with practices of southern India. This program became extremely popular here in the United States and in Europe, but, sadly, was canceled at the protest of a group of northern Ayurvedic doctors who claimed that marma therapy was dangerous. They cited that marmas were points to avoid—never to be touched, rubbed with pressure or used during therapy. This is just one example of the different Ayurvedic philosophies currently existing in the north and south of India.

Marma and Ayurvedic Massage

In most Western Ayurvedic massage books, marma point activation is described as a natural result of Ayurvedic massage. Marma points are part of the subtle-body system (see Chapter 3). There are 107 of these points, and they are considered to be subtle junctions between consciousness and matter. Enlivening these points with marma therapy is said to enhance the awareness of pure consciousness in the body. This awareness initiates a spontaneous healing response in the body at the deepest level of imbalance. Traditionally this very specific therapy was called *marma chikitsa.*

It is true that Ayurvedic massage will rub or press on marmas and offer a general stimulation of these points. In my training in marma therapy, these points were considered sacred, and their treatment had to be very specific. While massage will activate the marmas it will be too general to have a specific and desired therapeutic effect.

Marma points were first described on the battlefield in the south of India as points to protect. If a marma was injured or punctured in battle, the marma hit would describe the type and rate of one's death. As a result these points were traditionally avoided and their treatment was rare, highly safeguarded, and coveted.

In this book I will not delve into marma therapy as a part of Ayurvedic massage. This subject, according to my training, is a separate discipline, far too powerful and potentially harmful (if not administered correctly) to be considered as a part of massage therapy. I do introduce the treatments of two head marmas as a preparation for each Ayurvedic massage technique; however the entire subject of marma therapy is too extensive to be included here. Another volume in this series will reintroduce the marma and maha-marma program along with the five senses therapies I learned during my training in India.

Eight Branches of Ayurveda

Ayurveda is divided up into eight branches that complete its comprehensive approach to health care. Today, Ayurvedic students in one of the 250 colleges and universities in India usually choose a specialty, much as medical students do in America. The eight branches are: *Kayachikitsa* (internal medicine), *Shalakya Tantra* (ears, nose and throat), *Vishagara-vairodh Tantra* (toxicology), *Kaumara Bhritya* (pediatrics), *Shalya Tantra* (surgery), *Bhuta Vidya* (psychiatry), *Vajikarana* (aphrodisiacs), and *Rasayana* (rejuvenation). Of these, Rasayana and Vajikarana deal with the preservation of health and vigor, while the remaining branches deal primarily with the treatment of disease.[3]

In addition to the eight branches, there are over two thousand medicinal herbs classified in the Indian *Materia Medica* that are still in use today.[4] Ancient alchemists in the Ayurvedic tradition were extremely advanced for their time. The knowledge of how to prepare mercury, gold and other toxic metals to turn them into medicines was very sophisticated, as was turning minerals into a fine ash called *bhasma* that is easily absorbed into the bloodstream. Many of these preparations are used for reversal of the aging process and the attainment of full spiritual potential.

Charaka states, "Ayurveda is the knowledge that indicates the appropriate and inappropriate, happy or sorrowful conditions of living, what is auspicious or inauspicious for longevity, as well as the measure of life itself."[5] In Ayurveda, the measure of life is not determined by one's material wealth or political power but by a simple measure of contentment and spirituality. It is clear in *Charaka* that the main cause of disease is *pragya paradh* which means the "mistake of the intellect." Simply put, disease ensues when the intellect makes the ultimate mistake, when it starts to think of itself—the body and mind—as separate from the Divine or God itself. This separation breeds unfulfilling patterns of behavior and belief systems that ultimately manifest as physical or emotional disease. As a result, many of the Ayurvedic therapies, including massage, are focused on restoring the memory of pure consciousness in every cell of the body as well as on removing the disease.

The goal of an Ayurvedic prescription goes beyond good health and treatment of disease, into the direction of full human physical and spiritual potential. In fact, the foremost purpose of Ayurveda has always been to prepare for a spiritual process rather than to treat disease, and a successful spiritual process requires good physical health, a stable mind, and balanced subtle bodies. This concept will be explained in detail in Chapter 3.

Constitutional Analysis

In Ayurvedic medicine, prevention is dictated by the unique requirements of one's body type. Because we are unique, what we eat, how we exercise, when we sleep, and even where we prefer to live can all be understood according to our body type. There are three basic mind-body types that combine to make ten unique mind-body types. *Vata* types tend to be thin, hypermetabolic, and think and move quickly. They typically have dry skin and cold hands and feet. They do not like cold weather because they already have many of these cold, winter qualities inherent in their nature. I often refer to these types as Winter types. *Pitta* types are competitive, hot, and fiery with a medium frame. They prefer cool weather. Under some conditions they may get heartburn, skin rashes, inflammatory diseases, or they just burn out. They can be called Summer types. *Kapha* types are easy going and hypometabolic. They will hold on to more weight and water and tend to develop allergies and congestion.

They can become lethargic, obese, and even depressed under certain conditions. Kapha types mimic the properties of spring.

Understanding the body type of the patient is the hallmark of a preventive prescription, which might include diet, exercise, specific herbs, and seasonal cleansing techniques, including massage, that are all tailored to the patient's constitution.

Prevention

Ayurveda recognizes that all life—whether it be human, plant, or animal—must live in harmony with nature in order to survive. As the owner's manual of a car speaks of maintenance schedules for its long-term health, Ayurveda speaks of daily and seasonal routines called *dina charya* that insure maximal health and longevity. For example, birds fly south in the winter, as their survival depends on it. Leaves turn red and fall off trees in autumn—it's a law of nature. However, we tend to insulate ourselves from participating in the huge changes that take place from one season to the next even though our survival depends on it. Putting on or taking off a sweater and eating the same foods 365 days a year is an out-of-balance lifestyle, according to Ayurveda. In Ayurvedic medicine, prevention starts with a lifestyle that is in harmony with the changing cycles of nature.

Diet

We have made eating very complicated. There are more modern theories on eating than there are days in a month. While animals seem to balance their nutritional needs quite well with no knowledge of fats, proteins, or carbohydrates, we humans incessantly count calories and measure grams of fat only to find that the latest study tells us the rules of eating have changed once again. In Ayurveda the rules remain constant: as the seasons change and different foods and herbs are harvested, we naturally adjust our diets.

In winter, for example, squirrels eat nuts, a good source of protein and fat. This is a perfect food to help combat the cold, dry weather in the winter months (Vata season). Grains that are harvested in fall and cooked in winter are also a perfect Vata-balancing food. Cooked grains provide a warm, heavy nutritional base that helps us adapt to the cold of winter. In spring, after eating all the heavy nuts and grains during the long sedentary winter, nature again provides the perfect food. Light, leafy green veggies and berries are the first foods harvested in the spring (Kapha season) and are the natural antidote for the allergy season. These spring foods make up a Kapha-balancing or mucus-reducing diet. As the days get warmer in July and August, nature provides cooling fruits and vegetables to balance the heat of summer (Pitta season).

Ayurveda understands that the cycles of nature will provide what we need. These cycles also support a rhythm of life that is enjoyable. Unfortunately, our society has demanded that we rush, push, and shove our way through life in order to get ahead. One of the biggest social violations, according to Ayurveda, revolves around our meals. We frequently race through or, at times, even skip meals. Ayurveda recommends that the main meal be eaten at midday and that it be eaten slowly and calmly, much as it was a century or two ago. Crashing through our morning, racing through lunch, and coming home to eat the biggest meal of the day after 7:00 PM, when digestion and metabolism are winding down, could not be more against the powerful grain of Mother Nature.

Living in harmony with nature's cycles is a basic principle of Ayurveda and one that is still practiced today in many traditional cultures. Detailed information on Ayurvedic body types, diets, and seasonal and daily routines is available in my previous books, *The 3-Season Diet, Perfect Health for Kids,* and *Body, Mind, and Sport.*

Ayurvedic Diagnosis

Unlike a Western diagnosis, an Ayurvedic diagnosis begins by asking not *what is* the disease but rather *who has* the disease. It is not uncommon in Ayurveda, for example, to treat five people suffering from sleep disorders with five different herbs rather than one standard pill for insomnia. Remedies are formulated to treat the underlying cause of the condition in a particular individual rather than to treat a general class of symptoms.

In order to prescribe individualized treatments in this manner, Ayurvedic doctors must equip themselves with a different set of diagnostic tools. The Ayurvedic diagnosis starts with a thorough physical exam including inspection and palpation. The doctor begins by examining the seven tissues and the skin; then the "Nine Doors" (two eyes, two ears, two nostrils, mouth and throat, anus, and penis or vulva) are inspected and evaluated along with their secretions.[6] A detailed examination of the tongue gives a measure of the digestive state. Questions determine the timing of symptoms with reference to daily and seasonal cycles. The doctor takes histories and evaluates breath, heart, and joint sounds.

Pulse reading is one of the more common forms of Ayurvedic diagnosis. Some doctors prefer to diagnose only the pulse and to ask no questions of the patient before they begin their treatments. Reading the pulse determines the balance of the three doshas (Vata, Pitta, and Kapha) and their associated tissues and subtle energies. It is understood that if these three are in balance, the body will maintain a state of optimal health. The therapies are therefore aimed at restoring this balance rather than eradicating the disease. Ayurveda puts faith on the body's ability to heal itself, a sentiment shared by one of the world's more famous philosophers, Voltaire, who said, "The art of medicine consists of amusing the patient while Nature cures the disease."[7]

Ayurvedic Treatments

Ayurveda has numerous therapeutic modalities, massage being one that is highly regarded. Many of today's alternative therapies may have had their beginnings in Ayurveda. Aromatherapy, yoga therapy, herbology, sound and color therapies, detoxification therapies, acupuncture, exercise, meditation, breathing techniques, massage, and lifestyle modifications were all practiced thousands of years ago as a part of the Ayurvedic tradition. With the emphasis on dealing with the cause of disease, Ayurvedic doctors recommend many dietary and lifestyle changes as a means to remove habitual and causative factors. Once these changes have been made, the doctor will then typically prescribe a series of herbal treatments for the patient. The prescription can be simple, such as a single ground-up herb, or highly complex—a blend of fifty herbs. The Ayurvedic doctor may prescribe herbal compounds that can take days or weeks to prepare. Because of the sophisticated nature of most Ayurvedic preparations, the herbs perform clinically at a very high level without needing mega-dosages. If the patient has been living a toxic and non-spiritual lifestyle or is embarking on a spiritual path, the doctor may prescribe a series of cleansing or purification techniques called panchakarma, or "five actions of cleansing." These five actions include: *vamana* (emesis therapy), which removes mucus from the stomach; *virechana* (purgation therapy), where the liver, gallbladder, and skin are cleansed; *basti* (enema), which flushes the intestines; *rakta mokshana* (blood letting) to clean the blood; and medicated *nasya* (nasal oil inhalation).

Ayurvedic massage plays an important part in preparing for the cleansing actions of panchakarma. Without massage, the detoxification of panchakarma would be a long, harsh event rather than a luxurious treatment once reserved for royalty.

Panchakarma can last for a week and up to two or three months, with specific massage therapies each day. It is also prescribed as a primary tool for rejuvenation and longevity.

Western Ayurveda offers a comprehensive approach to health care with a set of therapeutic tools that understands and treats the relationship between body, mind, and spirit with great effectiveness. In these changing times we may find that yesterday's medicine is opening doors today for the enlightened doctors of tomorrow.

References

1.   David Frawley, *Ayurvedic Healing* (Salt Lake City, UT: Passage Press, 1989), p. xv.

2.   K.L. Bhishagratna, *Sushruta Samhita* (Varanasi, India: Chowkhamba Sanskrit Series Office, 1981), Vols. 1–2.

3.   Swami Sada Shiva Tirtha, *The Ayurvedic Encyclopedia* (Bayville, NY: Ayurvedic Health Center Press, 1998), p. 7.

4. James Duke, *Handbook of Medicinal Plants,* (Boca Raton, FL: CRC Press, 1986), Preface.

5. P.V. Sharma, *Charaka Samhita* (Varanasi, India: Chowkhamba Orientalia, 1981), Ch. 1, V-41.

6. Robert Svoboda, *Ayurveda: Life, Health, and Longevity* (New York, NY: Arkana Penguin Books, 1992), p. 177.

7. Robert Svoboda, *Ayurveda: Life, Health, and Longevity* (New York, NY: Arkana Penguin Books, 1992), p. 179–180.

Chapter Two

Introduction to Ayurvedic Massage

As part of the preparation process for panchakarma, Ayurvedic massage is considered a form of *snehana* or oleation, whereby the body can be treated either externally or internally with specific oils. This process promotes a softening of the impurities lodged deep in the body's cellular structure, loosening and making them available to be eliminated through the panchakarma techniques. When the snehana is administered externally through Ayurvedic massage it is called *bahya snehana*. There are numerous types of external snehana, or massage techniques, described in this book. Without an effective internal and external oleation process prior to panchakarma, the detoxification would be rendered less effective and, in some cases, even harmful to the body.

Fortunately, the menu of Ayurvedic massage therapies described in this volume can be administered outside of the panchakarma envelope with great success. In this book I am not teaching panchakarma therapies. Panchakarma is a series of eliminative and rejuvenative techniques that can be administered only by an Ayurvedic doctor. Ayurvedic treatments described in this book are powerful and can be offered alone or in a series without the guidance of an Ayurvedic doctor. These treatments can be performed by one or two Ayurvedic therapists working in synchrony. Two, three, and sometimes four of these therapies are linked together to complete an Ayurvedic treatment.

Introduction to the Ayurvedic Therapies

The following list summarizes the purpose and benefits of each therapy described in this book.

- *Garshana* treatments consist of a dry lymphatic skin brushing with either a wool or a silk glove. This "rubbing" increases heat and enhances circulation while exfoliating the skin so subsequent oil and herbal treatments can penetrate deeply into the freshly cleaned pores. This technique also produces static electricity, which alkalizes the blood and detoxifies the body.
- *Abhyanga,* the classic Ayurvedic massage, is an individually prepared herbal-oil massage designed to deeply penetrate the skin, relax the mind-body, break up impurities, and stimulate both arterial and lymphatic circulation, enhancing the delivery of nutrients to starved cells and the removal of stagnant waste. The desired result is a heightened state of awareness that will direct the internal healing system of the body.

  In addition, abhyanga begins to move the ten vayus, or subtle energies, in the body, which helps to remove the blocks in the nadis, allowing them to restore optimal function. Once the nadi paths are clear, healing and spiritual power can manifest in the body.
- *Vishesh* is a deep muscular Ayurvedic massage that breaks up adhesions and compromised circulation within the muscle spindles. When certain channels are blocked, then neither awareness nor blood can access deeply seated tissues. For certain body types and imbalances, this is an essential therapeutic approach.
- *Swedana* is an individually herbalized steam bath. The Ayurvedic swedana is unique because the head and the heart are kept cool during the steam bath while the body is heated to remove mental, emotional, and physical toxins lodged deeply within the tissues. The cool head and heart provide a sense of calm and openness while the therapeutic steam over the entire body can penetrate and cleanse deeply without the body becoming overheated and stressed.
- *Shirodhara* is administered by gently and methodically pouring warm herbalized oil over the forehead. This procedure synchronizes brain waves and profoundly coordinates and calms the mind, body, and spirit. While most Ayurvedic therapies have their impact

on the physical and energy sheaths of the subtle body system, shirodhara most effectively purifies the mental sheath, where patterns of behavior (*vasanas*) and emotional traumas can distract the mind from its role in supporting good health and spiritual growth.

- *Udvartana* is a deeply penetrating herbal paste lymphatic massage. This powerful exfoliating treatment magically conditions the skin while pressing stagnant lymphatic toxins out of the body. While mostly working on *rasa dhatu* (lymph) it enables the vayus to flow and activate the nadi system (see Chapter 3).
- The Ayurvedic facial, based on 5,000-year-old beauty secrets, aims to relax the mind while cleansing, nourishing and toning the skin. As the head, neck and face are where the nervous system is concentrated, treating these areas during an Ayurvedic facial has the ability to treat the entire nervous system. The facial is also a form of head massage activating powerful marmas, vayus, and nadis that balance all five sheaths of the subtle body system.

Ayurvedic Longevity

Ayurveda, as the "science of life," describes not only how to live your life but also how to make it last as long as possible. When we speak of longevity in the West we are usually talking about adding a few good years to our life. In ancient India, they were talking about extending life spans by fifty to a hundred years plus! During my training in India I was always fascinated by the topic of longevity and life extension. My Ayurvedic teachers spoke of ancient rejuvenation techniques that could totally transform the body of a withered ninety-year-old to that of a vibrant thirty-year-old. To them, these outrageous claims seemed strangely matter-of-fact. Neighboring countries also reported such life extension miracles. From a remote region in Tibet, the "five rites of rejuvenation" (a set of yoga exercises) have staked a recent claim to the fountain of youth. Stories about a British naval officer taking thirty or forty years off his body with Tibetan yoga techniques have made headlines here in the West.

Magic or Myth

I have heard stories of life extension ranging from one hundred to five hundred years using ancient Ayurvedic techniques. In India this notion of immortality, although somewhat hard to swallow by the skeptical West, seems alive and well. My favorite story is that of a Maharaj who reportedly lived to be 185 years old. As recounted in the book, *Maharaj,* by T.S. Murthy, Tapasviji Maharaj went through certain Ayurvedic rejuvenation therapies three times in order to extend his youthfulness to the ripe old age of 185. In these life extension treatments, or kya kalpa, the body was kept in isolation for three to six months. Aspirants would eat only rare herbs and medicated milk and receive a series of panchakarma longevity and Ayurvedic massage treatments each day. The treatments were hands-on rejuvenation techniques that purged the physiological stress and age out of the body's deep tissues. Developed in southern India, highly specific massage techniques were employed to balance the subtle bodies as well as to facilitate physiological detoxification. It was understood that to extend life successfully the treatments would need to be a transformation on the level of body, mind, and spirit. Subtle bodies, nadis, chakras, and vayus would all need to function in harmony in order to achieve this goal.

During the kya kalpa process, which is a form of cellular transformation, it is said that one's teeth and hair fall out and grow back new. Old skin sheds like a snake's, unveiling a new supple and youthful layer. On the ninety-first day of treatment one could expect improved eyesight, clarity of mind, and the strength and vigor of a thirty-year-old. Of course none of these reports have ever been documented to the satisfaction of Western science. However, the theories behind these practices are an interesting study, and could in fact provide us with a practical understanding of the long sought after fountain of youth, or, at the very least, good health.

Lost But Not Forgotten

In India there are still many Ayurvedic hospitals that use panchakarma therapies for the treatment of disease. Over the years these treatments have become known for physiological cleansing rather than for achieving longevity. No doubt they serve this purpose well, but when you are after the results of kya kalpa (life extension), cleansing alone will not serve your purpose. I have had these treatments in India on many occasions and have administered them for 16 years here in the United States. But only after numerous trips to India did I begin to understand some of the basic tenets of these treatments. For example, for the treatments to be successful:

- One had to have the ability to maintain absolute silence and seclusion in a deep meditative state for weeks or months at a time.
- One had to be in total control of all the senses at all times, which required a totally purified mind.
- One had to be physically strong enough to endure the process.

Although extreme, this didn't seem so much to ask considering a life extension benefit of fifty or sixty years. Even so, it was for this reason that the secrets of kya kalpa had been privy only to sages and monks who were capable of living these requirements as a way of life.

If these prerequisites seem beyond your personal reach or you are not interested in having your hair and teeth fall out and skin peel off, there is a slow but steady approach that is said to accomplish the elusive goal of life extension. In ancient times the kings and queens were given seasonal panchakarma and Ayurvedic massage treatments as a means to extend life and to safeguard the fair and just thinking required of the ruling class. A one-week series of panchakarma and Ayurvedic massage would actually instill the benefits of kya kalpa, and with successive treatments the benefits could be made permanent. In a way, they would transform the mind and awaken the spirit by Ayurvedically manipulating the physical body.

While panchakarma and kya kalpa techniques are administered only by an Ayurvedic doctor, the massage techniques and Ayurvedic therapies offered in this book as individual treatments are extremely effective in bringing the physical and subtle bodies back into harmony.

In fact, the mechanics of transformation of each aged cell, which result in life extension itself, are inherent in the Ayurvedic therapies described in this book. Each therapy sets up a specific internal environment that brings into co-existence two opposite forces, silence and activity, and establishes a powerful state of calm that triggers a dynamic physiological response. The best analogies for this process are to be found in the awesome forces of nature itself. A hurricane, for example, is a combination of gale force winds swirling around a still center. The bigger the silent eye of the hurricane, the more powerful the winds. This is the same law of nature we observe as tiny electrons spin around a nucleus and planets orbit a still sun. For us to harness this power and longevity we must be able to reproduce their environment inside of us: this is the goal of kya kalpa and panchakarma. As such, it should also be the goal of each Ayurvedic massage, and it starts with the intention of the therapist.

The success of these treatments is to a large degree dependent on the consciousness of the therapist. The reason each therapy is specially choreographed is that this allows the therapist not to be the "doer" of the therapy. When the therapist is doing the healing for the guest, the ego inevitably takes control, distracting the mind from the silence of the heart. The heart in Ayurveda is the source of both feelings and thoughts. During an Ayurvedic massage the mind is responding to the feelings of the heart and thinking only those thoughts initiated by the heart. If the mind is busy "fixing" the guest, the flow of consciousness from the heart is blocked as the mind takes control. When well grounded in the heart as the faculty of thought, the therapist connects to their own consciousness as the source of the therapy.

As we are all fundamentally expressions of consciousness, and as the cause of disease is the mind forgetting that we are sourced in consciousness, one of the goals of these therapies is to infuse the awareness into every cell of the guest. When the therapist taps into this experience of consciousness during a treatment, it stirs a corresponding awareness in the guest. When the guest becomes self-aware, their body can recognize the problem as a problem. From this place of deep silence there is nothing the body cannot heal.

These treatments act to initiate a self-healing response. The therapist is not a "healer" but one who enhances the ability of guests to heal themselves. The heightened internal awareness created from the state of silence triggers a cascade of spontaneous healings on a cellular level where we bury our stress, fears, and emotions.

Life Extension

When during a therapy the guest is taken into a deep, meditative state of silence, the basal metabolic rate is significantly lowered, and with successive treatment, it is lowered even more. If the body were a lake, it would become totally calm and crystal clear. In this state the body experiences itself more profoundly as a unified field of consciousness rather than thousands of physical parts.

Each Ayurvedic massage treatment provides deep relaxation as well as an experience of total luxury. The luxuriousness provides a calm that relaxes the body and gives access to the well protected storage sites of toxic tissues deep within the body. The cumulative effect of two and a half hours of such treatments for a week or more establishes an internal peace that remains as a hub of silence for all activity, and this immersion into inner silence allows the experience of consciousness to pervade every cell and become a way of life.

During Ayurvedic massage it is imperative for the therapist to create in the treatment room a cocoon of silence, beauty, and perfection. The treatments must be embarked upon with the intention not to heal pain with deeper massage pressure but to bring the guest's awareness into a state of silence so that they can be more self-aware and ultimately heal themselves.

When we talk of complete control of the senses as seen in the kya kalpa treatments, the process starts with a refinement of all the senses. It seems that throughout the course of evolution our senses have been sold a slightly bogus bill of goods. We have traded a world of unlimited human potential for a glitzier and sexier world, full of sensual pleasure and the pursuit of power. Originally, as infants we did not have access to our senses as we know them. They developed over time, and as they did, we became intoxicated with new sounds, tastes, colors, and shapes.

In Ayurveda the senses are considered avenues of consciousness that, in infancy, bring all the experiences of the outside world through the filter of the mind and directly to the heart as feelings. This is how mothers communicate with their babies without words for the first two years of life. It is a heart to heart level of communication based on feelings, and it doesn't get more direct. Even as adults the senses still make us feel. When you hear a favorite song, you feel good. When you smell a flower, you feel good. These feelings are heartfelt and are accessed via the five senses.

Typically our senses are so overloaded with external stimuli that they keep us from having a real experience of ourselves. The heart, which is the source of our feelings—and in Ayurveda is the source of all our thoughts, actions, and desires—is the ultimate eye of the hurricane, that calm center that supports all our mental, emotional, and physical activity.

Ayurvedic massage turns the senses inside out and makes us feel deeper parts of ourselves. It is human nature to protect ourselves from getting hurt emotionally, so we wall off the deep and delicate feelings of our hearts, making a mind-over-matter approach to life the norm. Certain Ayurvedic massage treatments transport awareness in the form of consciousness to the heart and then to every cell in the body. The heart, which is the source of both feelings and consciousness, is bombarded with this awareness, infusing feelings, consciousness, and healing into every cell. With this heightened state of self-awareness there is nothing that the body cannot fix. Instead of seeking happiness in the unreliable world of the relative, the senses provide access to the source of life and longevity itself. This is our own consciousness that we hold so very dear to our hearts.

During an Ayurvedic massage, it is said that if the therapist is experiencing a state of inner silence, then the treatment is better for the therapist than it is for the guest. For a treatment to be truly successful— meaning that it brings the guest to this silent state—their senses have to be surrounded by beauty and perfection, with every possible detail of their needs attended to.

Finally, it was traditionally required that the aspirant of kya kalpa have the strength and endurance to handle the experience. The traditional ninety-day kya kalpa treatments were drastically depleting prior to ultimate reward of rejuvenation. Panchakarma, because of the Ayurvedic massage, promises an experience of total rejuvenation. As I previously described, the senses make us aware of the eye of the hurricane located in the heart, while the lowering of the metabolic rate acts as a kind of calm lake where the body can see deeply and clearly into itself. The bigger the eye of the hurricane, the more powerful its wind— thus, the more energy is available to heal and rejuvenate the body from inside out. The experience of a series of panchakarma and Ayurvedic massage treatments establishes this rejuvenative calm on the level of each and every cell.

Chapter Three

Ayurvedic Massage and
the Subtle-Body System

In addition to physical detoxification and life extension, Ayurvedic massage carries an even more important purpose.

At conception, the subtle bodies, or fields of energy, of the new individual initiate the development of the embryo. These subtle bodies described in detail some five thousand years ago may be related to a new domain in science that measures heart fields—the electromagnetic fields radiating from the heart, through the body structure, and expanding some fifteen feet in diameter around the body. The subtle bodies encompass the physical body and subtle-energy fields that surround and infiltrate the body. Ayurvedic and yogic philosophy delineate this field into five subtle bodies or five sheaths, called *koshas*. The purpose of these five koshas is to support the development of the individual beginning at conception and continuing throughout their life, ultimately supporting their spiritual process.

Modern physics recognizes a unified field that pervades everything and out of which manifest all material expressions. Even the most subtle particles of matter like electrons and protons are just concentrated frequencies of the unified field. So at the root of every aspect of matter is a field vibrating at frequencies that correspond to its material expression. This field, according to Ayurveda, is our own consciousness. It is from this field that comes the creative spiritual life force (*shakti*) or love that fuels life itself.

After conception, the mother and child together create an electromagnetic field (heart field) that supports the progressive development of the subtle bodies into a healthy emotional and physical being. These sheaths of the subtle-body system develop around the source, pure consciousness, like the rings of an onion, from the most pure to the most gross.

The goal of Ayurveda and Ayurvedic massage is to prepare the koshas so they can facilitate the flow of consciousness and shakti through each of these fields, linking the grossest physical body with the most subtle field at the source of creation, called *Atman*. When the subtle bodies are balanced, then each sheath or kosha—including all aspects of mind, body, spirit, and emotions—can function up to its full harmonious potential. The following is a description of the five sheaths radiating from the center ring of the onion, consciousness, to the outermost layer, the physical body.

THE FIVE SUBTLE BODIES

At the center of this field is pure consciousness, the creative source from which everything comes. This is known as Atman.

The center field of pure consciousness is protected by the first subtle body known as *anandamaya kosha* or the sheath of bliss. Here the source itself, pure consciousness, merges with the power of this consciousness, *kundalini shakti,* from which comes the power to manifest a physical and emotional body. It is sometimes called the causal body because it causes the creation of the next four sheaths.

The second sheath is the sheath of intellect and discernment called the *vijnanamaya kosha*. The roles of this sheath include: pure intellect and understanding without emotion, the intrinsic knowledge of good and bad, and direct access to source. When the next three sheaths are balanced, one naturally chooses activities and makes decisions that are life supporting and in the direction of the bliss sheath or pure consciousness.

The third sheath, also called the great barrier sheath, is the mental sheath or *manomaya kosha*. This sheath of the mind contains desire, memories, ego, and emotion. It is here that we can become distracted by the mind and disconnected from access to the source.

The fourth sheath is the energy sheath or *pranamaya kosha*. This sheath regulates the flow of subtle energy in the body. It uses *prana* (subtle energy), the nadis (subtle nerve flow) and chakras (subtle-energy centers) to transform thought into action allowing the mind to affect and direct the body. It is here that many of the benefits of Ayurvedic massage are experienced.

The fifth sheath is the sheath of the gross or material body and is the *anna-maya kosha*. This kosha is the physical manifestation of the previous four subtle bodies and gives us our physical form. Through Ayurvedic massage, the physical sheath is purified allowing the energy sheath to begin purifying the mental sheath.

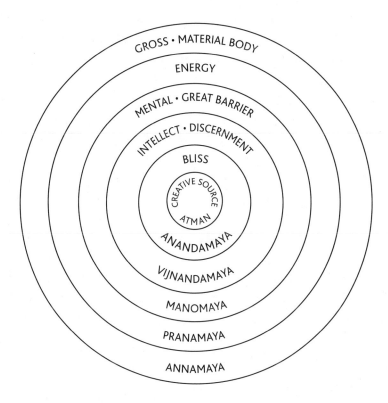

These five sheaths that begin with the source of consciousness and culminate with the manifestation of the physical body are created sequentially from the inside out, from the subtle to the material. The coherence and sanctity of the heart field, or subtle energetic bodies, are critical for the health, well-being, and spiritual process of the individual. The goal of the science of Ayurveda, Ayurvedic massage, and yoga is to support and balance the subtle bodies so that when an individual begins their spiritual life—no matter with what the discipline or religion—success will be insured. According to Vedic science, before one can enjoy all of the fruits of a spiritual life, physical health must be restored. The role of Ayurveda and massage is to restore optimal health as a preliminary goal before entering into a spiritual life. The sciences of both yoga and Ayurveda were created for this purpose — not only for physical health and longevity, but for the successful pursuit of a spiritual life and the achievement of our full potential as human beings.

Here in the West, we often utilize yoga as merely a physical and mental health tool and are often unaware that each posture carries a specific vibrational frequency designed to direct or redirect the subtle energy and pure consciousness fully and effectively through the five sheaths. Ayurveda and the achievement of perfect physical health prepare the body in order to support the spiritual process. Success is achieved when the mind gives up its need to be in control, the emotions free up their attachments to superficial pleasures and security, and the body is healthy enough to support optimal flow and movement of subtle energy through it. When this happens, the heart—which according to the *Yoga Vashistha* is the faculty of all thoughts, actions, and desires—becomes the holder of the reins. This means that the heart, or the consciousness within the heart, becomes the thinker of thoughts and as a result calls all the shots.

Effects of Ayurvedic Massage on the Annamaya Kosha (Physical Body)

The actual strokes of Ayurvedic massage affect primarily the physical body (annamaya kosha) and the energy body (pranamaya kosha). As described in Chapter 2 and in more detail later in this book, there are specific Ayurvedic massage treatments that will increase circulation, move lymph, break up scar tissue, or relieve muscle tension—all working on the physical body. With increased stress and tension the muscles constrict, and as a result less blood supply (and therefore oxygen) is available to maintain optimal function. If the stress persists over time, the muscles are forced to lay down a protective fibrous tissue (scar tissue) that does not require blood. Imagine if you did not water your lawn for a period of time. You would get crabgrass, which is a tougher version of grass, built on the fact that there is a less than ample water supply. When adequate blood supply is not available to the muscles, a tougher, non-elastic version of muscle is the result. Once the muscles begin accumulating fibrous tissue they become stiff and rigid. The ability of the muscle to contract smoothly is compromised, and it takes more effort to exercise or move the body. Soon inflexibility sets in creating structural problems as well as blocking the circulatory channels called srotas, which in turn block energy channels in the body, the vayus.

Ayurvedic massage activates the flow of Vata (wind), Pitta (bile), and Kapha (mucus), supporting the seven dhatus (bodily tissues) through a series of sixteen channels or srotas. It is through the sixteen srotas, the three doshas (Vata, Pitta, and Kapha), and seven dhatus that Ayurvedic massage primarily works on the physical body or annamaya kosha.

THE SIXTEEN SROTAS

The first three srotas control the flow of water, food, and breath to the body.

1. *Pranavaha srotas* carry prana (breath and life force) to the circulatory and respiratory system.
2. *Annavaha srotas* carry food from the digestive and assimilative channels.
3. *Ambhuvaha srotas* regulate water metabolism.

The next seven srotas support each of the major tissues or *dhatus* of the body.

4. *Rasavaha srotas* carry plasma (*rasa*) and lymph.
5. *Raktavaha srotas* carry blood (*rakta*).
6. *Mamsavaha srotas* supply the muscular system.

7. *Medavaha srotas* nourish fat cells.
8. *Asthivaha srotas* nourish the skeletal system (bones).
9. *Majjavaha srotas* nourish the nervous system and marrow.
10. *Shukravaha srotas* supply the reproductive system.

The next three srotas are in charge of removing waste from the body.

11. *Swedavaha srotas* carry sweat.
12. *Purishavaha srotas* carry feces.
13. *Mutravaha srotas* carry urine.

The next srotas are channels that carry thought—originating in the heart and connecting with the mind.

14. *Manovaha srotas* carry thought from the mental system.

Two more channels exist for carrying menstrual fluid and lactate.

15. *Artavavaha srotas* carry menstrual fluid.
16. *Stanyavaha srotas* carry breast milk and lactation channels.

Effects of Ayurvedic Massage on the Pranamaya Kosha (Energy Sheath)

Once the physical body has been relieved of gross tension, adequate blood supply has been restored to the musculoskeletal system, and all the srotas are functional, the effects of Ayurvedic massage naturally impact the pranamaya kosha or energy sheath. Here on this level, the intricacy of each Ayurvedic massage stroke moves energy (vayus, nadis, and chakras) in the pranamaya kosha. There are nearly a hundred different Ayurvedic massage strokes described in this book that uniquely move subtle energy in the body. In this sheath, once the flow of oxygen and blood supply are re-established and the three doshas (Vata, Pitta, and Kapha) are flowing through the srotas in the annamaya kosha (physical sheath), the ten individual pranas that are more commonly known as the "ten vayus" can begin to function on the subtle-energy level of the body. These ten vayus move energy throughout the body traveling through non-physical channels called nadis. There are 72,000 nadis in the body that, like meridians, cover most every corner of the human body. Of the 72,000 nadis described, thirty-six are commonly discussed, and only six of these nadis carry kundalini shakti—the spiritual force that is constantly moving toward its goal on the top of the subtle-body system (the crown).[1] Interestingly, the nadis manifest in the physical body only when they are activated by a moving vayu or energy; thus they exist in both the annamaya and pranamaya koshas. Most activities will move one or more of the ten vayus, thus activating a nadi. Depending on the nature of an activity, the vayus can be moved in a positive or negative direction. As a result, not all nadis when activated by the vayus will elicit a positive effect in the body. Their impact can be on a physical, mental, emotional, or spiritual plane—either positive or negative. Without optimal flow of the vayus, the physical body will suffer, creating a foothold for disease (described later) in the same way that imbalance in the physical body will disturb the vayu flow in the pranamaya kosha.

The Ten Vayus
The ten vayus rule in the house of Vata. The first five vayus are called the sub-doshas of Vata, controlling major Vata functions. The second five vayus control minor functions.

Prana—considered the vayu most connected to the life force. It moves from heart to head via the respiratory system and controls breathing, circulation, mental stability, thoughts, and feelings.

Udana—located in the throat, it controls the speech centers. It represents an upward moving vayu that transforms feelings into words. If udana is blocked it will affect the eyes, ears, nose, throat, head, and neck. Blockages here can mimic the mental dysfunction seen in blocked prana vayu.

Samana—balancing the upward and downward flow of the vayus. It is the air that the digestive system needs to burn. It is the nervous system's relation to the digestive system and as a result can cause stress-related eating disorders and digestive disturbances. Samana is responsible for distributing food or fuel to the cells of the body and brain. It uses channels of rasa (lymph) and rakta (blood) to nourish both the physical body and the flow of subtle energy (vayus) through the nadis into the chakras.

Apana—the downward moving force that controls elimination, reproduction, and the power moving into the pelvis and lower extremities. Blockages here can disturb sexual function and eliminative processes. It is closely related to prana vayu and as a result is connected to brain centers. Weakness in apana can deplete prana and vice-versa. Chronic mental stress can call on apana for support and create patterns of dysfunction in the brain that create imbalance in apana.

Vyana—controls the whole body. It depends on the balanced function of the first four vayus to function properly. It controls the circulatory system, nerve flow, muscles, and joints. It creates a normal field of energy around the body. When vyana vayu is blocked a more severe imbalance can usually be detected.

Note: These imbalances in the vayus (as well as in Pitta and Kapha) are described, diagnosed, and treated in detail in my Pulse Diagnosis tape series.

Minor Vayus

Kurma Vayu—controls blinking, governed by apana.

Naga Vayu—controls vomiting and belching, governed by samana.

Devadatta Vayu—controls yawning and sleep, governed by prana and the heart.

Krikara Vayu—controls sneezing, governed by udana.

Dhananjaya Vayu—controls swelling and decomposition of the body, governed by vyana.

Effects of Ayurvedic Massage on the Nadi System

The nadi system will function only if the associated vayus are flowing. The vayus, of course, will flow normally only if the srotas are moving gracefully through the annamaya kosha. Ayurvedic massage will first impact the body on a physical level, then as the more dense physical levels become balanced, the subtle levels can become functional. Normally functioning srotas balance Vata, Pitta, and Kapha, which support normally functioning vayus, which support normally functioning nadis. Only when all of the above are functional can the chakras begin to move kundalini shakti up the spine to the goal of the subtle-body system—the *bindu* point on the crown of the head.

There are only six nadis that carry kundalini shakti on its journey from the first chakra in the pelvis to the bindu point. Not all of these nadis actually reach the goal. Some of the kundalini-carrying nadis are complete and others are non-culminating nadis. The exact nadi the kundalini shakti chooses has a great impact on one's spiritual life, mental and emotional health, and physical well-being. The more balanced the subtle bodies, srotas, doshas, vayus, and supportive nadis (see following text) are prior to a kundalini arousal—say, as a child—the more direct the chosen nadi will be.

- *Brahmi* nadi: quick complete rising—most rare.
- *Chitrini* nadi: direct, complete rising.
- *Lakshmi* nadi: deflected and dangerous rising—not complete.
- *Vajra* nadi: starts in 2nd chakra—deflected not complete.
- *Saraswati* nadi: deflected rising—not complete.
- *Susumna* nadi: stable and preferred rising.[1]

There are fourteen main nadis that provide subtle-energy balance to the body that are actively treated with Ayurvedic massage. Some of these nadis have additional roles in the subtle-body system that are critical to spiritual development. For this discussion, I will mention only their impact on the physical and energy bodies in relation to Ayurvedic massage.

- *Ida* and *pingala* nadis wrap up the spine, bring prana through the sinuses, and regulate the sense of smell.
- *Sankhini* and *payasvini* nadis regulate hearing.
- *Gandhari* and *pusha* nadis regulate sight.
- *Hastijihva* and *yashasvati* nadis regulate movement of the limbs.
- *Saraswati* nadi, in addition to carrying kundalini, regulates taste.
- *Visvodhara* nadi regulates the digestive system.
- *Kuhu* nadi regulates the reproductive and urinary tract systems.
- *Varuna* nadi regulates respiration, circulation, and touch.
- *Alambusha* nadi regulates elimination.
- *Susumna* nadi, in addition to carrying kundalini shakti, regulates the nervous system.

Effects of Ayurvedic Massage on the Chakra System

Also in the energy sheath, or pranamaya kosha, are the six chakras or areas associated with six spinal levels in which the nadis are concentrated. On the physical plane, or annamaya kosha, the chakras are represented by a concentration of glands and nerve plexuses. The word "chakra" means a "wheel" that is spun and energized by the movement of vayus through a concentrated field of nadis. In fact many so-called kundalini experiences are just the sensation of moving vayus rather than a true spiritual experience. There are six chakras that are activated by the movement of vayus and nadis that are arranged from gross to subtle much as the subtle bodies or sheaths in which they reside. The lower chakras represent functions that regulate physical activities (lower functions) and the upper chakras regulate more subtle (higher) functions.

The Six Chakras

Muladhara chakra—located in the perineum, root, or anal area, it is governed by the earth element and is the keeper of the kundalini shakti until it begins its journey upward.

Svadhisthana chakra—governed by the water element and located in the genital region, it controls reproduction.

Manipura chakra—found in the navel area, it is governed by the fire element and controls the connection to the cosmos.

Anahata chakra—governed by air element, it is located in the heart center and controls the sacred heart or the connection to pure consciousness.

Vishuddha chakra—located at the throat center and governed by the element of space, it regulates the connection between mind and body.

Ajna chakra—located between the eyebrows, it is governed by the mind and awareness and purifies the subtle bodies.

Sahasrara—often called the crown or seventh chakra, it is not exactly a chakra. It is called the thousand-petal lotus, and it is the goal of the kundalini shakti on its journey from the muladhara chakra. Once kundalini shakti reaches sahasrara, it activates all the brain centers to make its final ascent to the *brahmarandhra*—the twelve-petal lotus on top of the thousand-petal lotus and the pinnacle or bindu.

Just as the shakti has a goal to move from the inner sheath (anandamaya kosha) to the outer sheath (annamaya kosha) of the subtle bodies, it also has a goal to move from the first chakra in the pelvis (muladhara) to the thousand-petal lotus (sahasrara) on the top of the head and ultimately the bindu point atop the brahmarandhra.

Ayurvedic massage plays an important part in this process. In most people, stress has created such tension in the physical body that the srotas, doshas, and vayus have also become stagnant and constricted. If the vayus are not moving, there is no nadi activation or chakra stimulation, and as a result there is poor physical and mental health and no spiritual progress. If the vayus are stagnant, this will result in physical imbalance. For example if apana vayu (which is the downward flowing vayu) is blocked, there may be difficulty conceiving a child, or one could be chronically constipated. If prana or udana vayus (upward flowing vayus) are blocked, then clarity of thought and mental stability may be affected.

Vayus must be moved in the proper direction and in the appropriate manner. As previously mentioned, vayu activation can do as much harm as good depending on the kind of movement and the type of activity.

The state of balance and harmony of the subtle bodies, vayus, nadis, and srotas, as well as the mental body, are considered to be determining factors in which nadi pathway the kundalini shakti will take on its journey to bindu. Each of the six different nadi risings will have its own obstacles and therefore predispositions to certain mental, emotional, and physical imbalances. Prior to reaching bindu, some of the non-culminating risings will give flashy spiritual experiences along the way. Many of these spiritual experiences, however, are often just glimpses— where a nadi takes the kundalini shakti to a fairly high rising but not to completion. Here, from a distant view of the goal, the seeker may have inconsistent, dramatic spiritual experiences that are neither permanent nor authentic.[1] Many of these non-culminating risings give spiritual powers and experiences that often distract the seeker from completing the journey. It is only upon reaching the *makara* point (just above the brow or ajna chakra) in a culminating rising on the final ascent to bindu that one experiences a true spiritual process, according to the ancient science of Kundalini Vidya.[1]

In this regard, Ayurvedic massage plays an important role in the physical, mental, and spiritual well-being of the individual. How well balanced the subtle-body system is prior to the first kundalini arousal during childhood will determine which of the six nadis is chosen. This is why, in traditional India, infant massage is considered an absolute must for new mothers to perform on their children. These strokes nourish the subtle bodies, preparing the child for the most direct rising of the kundalini. A good and direct rising not only means that the child will have a fruitful spiritual life, it means that the physical, mental, and energy bodies will be harmonious, and the child will enjoy a healthy, prosperous, and long life. In the same way that the subtle-body system of infants is affected, adults can experience the benefits of Ayurvedic massage.

Effects of Ayurvedic Massage on the Manomaya Kosha (Mental Sheath)

The next more subtle sheath, the manomaya kosha (mental sheath), is dependent on the proper functioning of the physical and energy sheaths to support balanced mental activity. As mentioned, if the upward moving vayus are not balanced, then mental function will be altered. Altered mental function can create belief systems and patterns of behavior that are protective, defensive, and dangerous to the subtle bodies or spiritual process. These patterns of defensive behavior create reactive emotions that lodge fear in the limbic system (emotional cortex) of the brain. The emotional constrictions create desires (often unhealthy) called vasanas that drive us into activities that will move the vayus in an unhealthy direction. Thus the emotions carried by these vasanas find themselves lodged in the physical sheath, needing Ayurvedic massage to be released. Dr. Candace Pert wrote a groundbreaking book called *The Molecules of Emotion* in which she proved that emotional neurotransmitters of the brain do in fact find themselves lodged in the physical body—a theory that was understood in Vedic philosophy thousands of years ago.

Let's recap this process. The stress and tension that are so common in our daily life create constricted muscles and blood vessels that block srotas (channels) and stagnate the function of Vata, Pitta, and Kapha (doshas) in the physical sheath. This compromises the movement of the ten vayus, affecting the function of the both the physical sheath (annamaya kosha) and energy sheath (pranamaya kosha). Without balanced vayu function, physical and mental health can be compromised. In addition, compromised vayu function will block the nadis involved in chakra activation and spiritual progress. Imbalanced flow of vayus, due to inappropriate activities, will activate certain nadis that create disharmony in the mental sheath (manomaya kosha). When the mental sheath is imbalanced, vasanas, or desires, are created that drive one to do activities that harm the function of the vayus and once again aggravate the ten vayus of the energy sheath, resulting in further stagnation in the physical sheath. Srotas and doshas become imbalanced, and the body becomes ill.

Ayurvedic massage will greatly help the function of the physical body and the movement of the srotas, doshas, vayus, and nadis in the physical and energy sheaths but has little impact on the mental sheath—the mind and emotions. Certain Ayurvedic techniques like head massage, marma therapy, and particularly shirodhara (which is the pouring of warm oil over the forehead) have a dramatic impact on releasing old beliefs lodged in the limbic system of the brain. With consecutive treatments of shirodhara, even the most advanced and deep seated vasanas can be addressed. In some cases shirodhara can be prescribed daily for three to six months—of course, under a doctor's supervision. This is a very powerful therapy that can take your guests to an entirely new state of self-awareness.

In the mental sheath there are other types of deep seated stress called *samskaras*. Samskaras are impressions or patterns of thought that could be due to chronic physical stress and imbalance using the pathways just described. Samskaras can also be very old stressors that create patterns of behavior and thought that are carried in the mental sheath (manomaya kosha) for lifetimes. The mental sheath is called the great barrier sheath because of the difficult to unravel samskaras. These samskaras are lodged deeply in the nervous system, and the longer they remain in place, the deeper the canyon of the engagement, and the more difficult they are to remove. Unless the nervous system is disarmed—in other words, convinced that it is safe enough to open its protective gates—these samskaras and associated patterns of behavior will stay in place for lifetimes. Ayurvedic treatments like panchakarma and kya kalpa are designed to disarm the nervous system and access the source of these samskaras. Shirodhara can also have this effect if the treatment is done effectively as I will describe later in this book.

Recently, we had a guest named Jenny who was receiving sshirodhara, and during the treatment she went steadily deeper and deeper. In this procedure the metabolic rate drops, and the brain waves become slow and coherent. The state of calm achieved with shirodhara is unparalleled by other relaxation techniques, and it brings the nervous system into the depths of inner silence. Suddenly, about three-quarters of the way through a forty-minute shirodhara session, Jenny's whole body jumped. Normally guests jerk as they lower themselves into the stillness but rarely once they get really deep. From the depths of her being, Jenny jerked so hard she almost rose off the table. That night she was awakened by the same intense jerk of her entire body. This time she remembered the dream that triggered it. She told me that the day she jumped while on the shirodhara table she was reliving the pain of the knee replacement surgery she had had. The pain was so bad she said that she just blocked it out, and it wasn't until her nervous system was completely disarmed by the shirodhara that she was able to move through the old trauma.

Pain and Bliss

In Ayurveda pain has a specific purpose in the body. Pain is said to be the direct opposite of bliss or pure consciousness. The purpose of the pain is to bring the body's awareness *to* the pain and then *through* the pain to establish itself in the bliss. Let's say the body is deeply settled and the protective nervous system is disarmed during a shirodhara or a two-person Ayurvedic massage. In this deep stillness the nervous system becomes aware of any stress or strain that inhibits the flow of stillness into every cell of the body. Naturally the body will move its attention to the pain or strain and, if all goes well, move through this pain to establish a new awareness of self at a deeper level of stillness. The goal is to have this pure experience of consciousness in every cell of the body—moving pure consciousness from the bliss sheath (anandamaya kosha) to the physical sheath (annamaya kosha). When this happens, the chakras and nadis can carry the kundalini shakti up the spine to its goal—the bindu point on the top of the chakra system. This process cannot be completed unless the physical, energy, and mental sheaths are balanced, stable, and functioning in harmony.

The next sheath is the vijnanamaya kosha, the intellectual or discernment sheath. This is where one has the ability to choose without the drive of imbalanced vasanas and the habit of deeply seated samskaras. If the mental sheath is not balanced, then the pull of the old vasanas and samskaras will distract the mind in the discernment sheath from being able to choose wisely in the direction of spirituality. With an unpurified mental sheath, choices will be in the direction of supporting the status quo set up by the old, deep seated patterns of behavior. Once the mental sheath is cleared, the individual mind can choose, without distraction, to move into the bliss sheath or anandamaya kosha. Once the bliss sheath is activated, the flow of shakti and consciousness can freely move through each kosha creating better health, peace of mind, and spiritual progress throughout one's life.

Ayurvedic massage and some of the therapies described in this book play a very important role in purifying the subtle-body system. As you can see, if the subtle bodies, doshas, vayus, nadis, chakras, and srotas are blocked, then physical imbalance, emotional disturbance, and mental unrest will be the accepted human condition (which it is in our current society). The goal of this book is to introduce Ayurvedic massage techniques that, while steeped in tradition, will unravel stressors on both the subtle and physical levels that will effectively put your guests on the road to permanent spiritual and physical well-being.

Note: The emphasis of these introductory chapters is not on the fundamentals and details of Ayurveda. For that many textbooks exist. My purpose in these chapters is to share the actual pathways Ayurvedic massage uses to treat the body holistically, addressing in the most powerful way possible the human body, mind, and spirit.

1.   The most comprehensive and well written resource describing the subtle-body system is a book called *Kundalini Vidya: The Science of Spiritual Transformation* by Joan Harrigan, Ph.D. It can be purchased through www.kundalinicare.com or by calling (865) 531–2004.

Chapter Four

Ayurvedic Massage According to Body Type

Before giving an Ayurvedic massage, it is important to understand a little about your guest's constitution or body type. As described in Chapter 1, there are three governing principles or doshas in Ayurvedic medicine: Vata (wind/winter), Pitta (bile/summer), and Kapha (mucus/spring). Dosha means impurity, and these three doshas are the first physical manifestation of the body from the unmanifest field of pure consciousness or pure energy. Thus they are impure only because they are the first deviation from the field of absolute purity from which everything comes.

In previous books, I have described the body type principles in relation to their associated seasons. Winter, which is cold and dry, relates to the Vata body type, which is also cold and dry. Both winter and Vata are governed by air or wind. Air moves quickly and easily, and therefore Vata controls movement in the body. Summer, which is a season of heat, relates to the body type Pitta. Both are governed by fire, and in the body, Pitta is in charge of metabolic activities like digestion, manufacturing and breaking down biochemicals, and skin function. Spring, which is a wet, rainy, and muddy time of year, relates to the Kapha body type. Both spring and Kapha are governed by earth and water, which control structural function and the lubricating activities of the body.

These three basic types combine to form a total of ten types:

Vata = Winter

Pitta = Summer

Kapha = Spring

Vata - Pitta

Pitta - Vata

Pitta - Kapha

Kapha - Vata

Kapha - Pitta

Vata - Pitta - Kapha

Vata - Kapha

For the purposes of an Ayurvedic massage it is helpful for the therapist to know the guest's body type in order to choose appropriate treatment times, herbs, and oils for that constitution. The following are some distinct characteristics of each of the three main types.

Characteristics of Vata (Winter) Type

Light, thinner build

Performs activity quickly

Tendency toward dry skin

Aversion to cold weather

Irregular hunger and digestion

Quick to grasp new information, also quick to forget

Tendency toward worry

Tendency toward constipation

Tendency toward light and interrupted sleep

Characteristics of Pitta (Summer) Type

Moderate build

Performs activity with medium speed

Aversion to hot weather

Prefers cold food and drinks

Sharp hunger and strong digestion

Can't skip meals

Medium time to grasp new information

Average memory

Tendency toward reddish hair and complexion, moles, and freckles

Good public speakers

Tendency toward irritability and anger

Enterprising and sharp in character

Characteristics of Kapha (Spring) Type

Solid, heavier build

Greater strength

Greater endurance, slow and methodical in activity

Oily, smooth skin

Slow digestion, mild hunger

Tranquil, steady personality

Slow to grasp new information, slow to forget

Slow to become excited or irritated

Sleep is heavy and long

Hair is plentiful, thick, and wavy

As each body type drifts out of balance there are certain tell-tale signs and symptoms that will signal the therapist of a Vata, Pitta, or Kapha imbalance. Each Ayurvedic massage technique in this book has indications with regard to its effectiveness for Vata, Pitta, and Kapha. Diagnosing and treating imbalances is not in the scope of practice for an Ayurvedic massage therapist, nor is it the intention of this book. However, I do think it is important for an Ayurvedic massage therapist to have a basic understanding of balance and imbalance according to Ayurvedic principles.

Classic Symptoms of Vata (Winter) Types

Dry or rough skin

Insomnia

Constipation

Fatigue

Headaches

Intolerance of cold

Underweight or losing weight

Anxiety, worry, and restlessness

Attention Deficit with Hyperactivity Disorder

Classic Symptoms of Pitta (Summer) Types

Rashes

Inflammatory skin conditions (including acne)

Stomach aches

Diarrhea

Controlling and manipulative behavior

Visual problems or burning in the eyes

Excessive body heat

Hostility, irritability

Excessive competitive drive

Classic Symptoms of Kapha (Spring) Types

Oily skin

Slow digestion

Sinus congestion

Nasal allergies

Asthma

Obesity

Skin growths

Possessiveness, neediness

Apathy

Depression

Spaciness

Difficulty paying attention

Constitutional Analysis

Prior to an Ayurvedic massage or therapy it is a valuable to give the guest an Ayurvedic body type assessment tool. Once the tool is completed, the therapist will have a better sense of which therapy is most appropriate. An assessment tool will not finish the process for body type determination. To accurately determine the body type, a physical exam, interview, and pulse diagnosis by an Ayurvedic practitioner are needed.

The body type assessment tool that follows will tell the therapist which dosha is currently predominant. How much of the predominating dosha is a result of body type factors and how much is due to an imbalance of that dosha is not a function of the assessment tool. For the therapist, treating the predominant dosha will treat both the imbalance and body type in a more general but still therapeutic fashion.

On the assessment tool, ask the guest to circle the descriptions that most suit them. If two or all three qualities accurately describe them, then circle them all. If none of the qualities apply then leave that section blank.

MENTAL PROFILE

	WINTER	SUMMER	SPRING
Mental activity	Quick mind, restless	Sharp intellect agressive	Calm, steady, stable
Memory	Short-term best	Good general memory	Long-term best
Thoughts	Constantly changing	Fairly steady	Steady, stable, fixed
Concentration	Short-term focus best	Better than average mental consentration	Good ability for long-term focus
Ability to learn	Quick grasp of learning	Medium to moderate grasp	Slow to learn new things
Dreams	Fearful, flying, running, jumping	Angry fiery, violent, adventurous	Include water, clouds, relationships, love
Sleep	Interrupted, light	Sound, medium	Sound, heavy, long
Speech	Fast sometimes missing words	Fast, sharp, clear-cut	Slow, clear, sweet
Voice	High pitch	Medium pitch	Low pitch
Mental Subtotal			

BEHAVIORAL PROFILE

	WINTER	SUMMER	SPRING
Eating speed	Quick	Medium	Slow
Hunger level	Irregular	Sharp, needs food when hungry	Can easily miss meals
Food and drink	Prefers warm	Prefers cold	Prefers dry and warm
Achieving goals	Easily distracted	Focused and driven	Slow and steady
Giving/donations	Gives small amounts	Gives nothing, or large amounts infrequently	Gives regularly and generously
Relationships	Many casual	Intense	Long and deep
Sex drive	Variable or low	Moderate	Strong
Works best	While supervised	Alone	In groups
Weather preference	Aversion to cold	Aversion to heat	Aversion to damp, cool
Reaction to stress	Excites quickly	Medium	Slow to get excited
Financial	Doesn't save, spends quickly	Saves, but big spender	Saves regularly accumulates wealth
Friendships	Tends toward short-term friendships, make friends quickly	Tends to be a loner friends related to occupation	Tends to form long-lasting friendships
Behavioral Subtotal			

EMOTIONAL PROFILE

	WINTER	SUMMER	SPRING
Moods	Changes quickly	Changes slowly	Steady, unchanging
Reacts to stress with	Fear	Anger	Indifference
More sensitive to	Own feelings	Not sensitive	Others' feelings
When threatened, tends to	Run	Fight	Make peace
Relations with spouse/parents	Clingy	Jealous	Secure
Expresses Affection	With words	With gifts	With touch
When feeling hurt	Cries	Argues	Withdraws
Emotional trauma causes	Anxiety	Anger	Depression
Confidence level	Timid	Outwardly self-confident	Inner confidence
Emotional Subtotal			

PHYSICAL PROFILE

	WINTER	SUMMER	SPRING
Amount of hair	Average	Thinning	Thick
Hair type	Dry	Normal	Oily
Hair color	Light brown, blonde	Red, auburn	Dark brown, black
Skin	Dry, rough or both	Soft, normal to oily	Oily, moist, cool
Skin temperature	Cold hands/feet	Warm	Cool
Complexion	Darker	Pink-red	Pale-white
Eyes	Small	Medium	Large
Whites of eyes	Blue/brown	Yellow or red	Glossy white
Size of teeth	Very large or very small	Small-medium	Medium-large
Weight	Thin, hard to gain	Medium	Heavy, gains easily
Elimination	Dry, hard, thin easily constipated	Many during day, soft to normal	Heavy, slow, thick, regular
Resting pulse			
Men	70–90	60–70	50–60
Women	80–100	70–80	60–70
Veins and tendons	Very prominent	Fairly prominent	Well covered
Physical Subtotal			

FITNESS PROFILE

	WINTER	SUMMER	SPRING
Exercise tolerance	Low	Medium	High
Endurance	Fair	Good	Excellent
Strength	Fair	Better than Average	Excellent
Speed	Very good	Good	Not so fast
Competition	Doesn't like competitive pressure	Driven competitor	Deals easily with competitive pressure
Walking speed	Fast	Average	Slow and steady
Muscle tone	lean, low body fat	Medium, with good definition	Brawny/bulky, with high fat percentage
Runs like	Deer	Tiger	Bear
Body size	Small frame, lean or long	Medium frame	Large frame, fleshy
Reaction time	Quick	Average	Slow
Fitness Subtotal			

TOTALS

	WINTER	SUMMER	SPRING
Mental			
Behavioral			
Emotional			
Physical			
Fitness			
Body Type Totals			

Once all the profiles are tallied, then choose the body type with the highest score: Vata, Pitta, or Kapha. If two body type scores are similar then both doshas are predominating. In this case, make dosha modifications that reflect both body type and season. For example, if the score is Vata 21, Pitta 25, Kapha 13, the working body type is Pitta-Vata. If this therapy is in January, which is in the Vata Season, then choose the Vata modifications for this guest.

If the score is Vata 15, Pitta 14, Kapha 26, the working body type is Kapha. When the result is conclusively one body type, as in this example, then treat the body type without adjusting for the season. Treatment modifications here would be for Kapha.

Body Type Modifications

Based on body type results, the following modifications to the massage oil can be made for Vata, Pitta, or Kapha body types.

Essential Oils

Essential oils can be added to the massage oil. Twenty to thirty drops of oil, or up to a 5% dilution, can be added to one cup of Ayurvedic massage oil.

Vata Essential Oils

Basil

Fennel

Marjoram

Orange

Geranium

Bergamot

Benzoin

Cardamom

Cinnamon

Pitta Essential Oils

Sandalwood

Lavender

Lemon

Ylang Ylang

Chamomile

Peppermint

Fennel

Rose

Neroli

Melissa (Lemon Balm)

Kapha Essential Oils

Rosemary

Eucalyptus

Camphor

Frankincense

Clary Sage

Juniper

Myrrh

Black Pepper

Clove

Tri-Doshic Essential Oils

Rose

Jasmine

Lavender

Sandalwood

Frankincense

Melissa (Lemon Balm)

Ginger

Fennel

AYURVEDIC MASSAGE BASE OILS

	VATA	PITTA	KAPHA
Sesame	Balances	Aggravates	Neutral
Olive	Balances	Not indicated	Not indicated
Almond	Balances	Aggravates	Aggravates
Castor	Balances	Aggravates	Not indicated
Coconut	Aggravates	Balances	Aggravates
Sunflower	Neutral	Balances	Not indicated
Ghee	Balances	Balances	Aggravates
Mustard	Balances	Aggravates	Balances
Corn	Aggravates	Aggravates	Balances

Sesame Oil

Classically, sesame is the oil of choice for Ayurvedic massage. Ayurvedic doctors will use sesame oil for most imbalances by medicating it with herbs. The properties of sesame oil are:

Heavy

Sweet

Bitter

Astringent

Heating

Balances Vata

Increases Pitta

Neutral for Kapha

Certain essential oils can be added to the sesame oil to enhance or adjust its properties as previously described.

Traditionally, herbs are cooked into the sesame oil to accentuate its medicinal properties. The process is elaborate and does not fall within the scope of this book. Herbal oils can be purchased pre-made from Ayurvedic supply houses. The most common therapeutic Ayurvedic oils are:

Amla Oil: Sesame oil cooked with the herb Amalaki—balances Pitta and Vata.

Bhringaraj Oil: Sesame oil cooked with the herb Bhringaraj—balances Pitta and Vata.

Brahmi Oil: Pure brahmi oil is available, and it is good for Vata and Pitta. Brahmi balances the mind and the senses by increasing circulation to the brain. It is classically used for improving memory, sleep disorders, and focusing ability. Mixed with coconut oil it balances Pitta. Mixed with sesame oil it balances Vata.

Chandan Oil: Sesame oil cooked with sandalwood. It is beneficial for Pitta primarily but is also therapeutic for Vata and Kapha. It treats inflammatory conditions as well as balancing the mind.

Dashamula Oil: Sesame oil mixed with dashamula [ten roots—ashwaganda, yasti mudha (licorice), punarnava, kumari (aloe vera), shatavari, vidari, bala, bilva, arjuna, goksura]. This oil provides deep rejuvenation for Vata and cleansing for Kapha.

Mahanarayan Oil: Sesame oil and castor oil cooked with ashwaganda, shatavari, bilva, and bala. It is classically used for musculoskeletal aches and pains. It balances Vata and Kapha.

Neem Oil: Sesame oil cooked with neem. It balances Pitta predominantly and is used to treat chronic skin conditions.

Vacha Oil: Sesame oil cooked with vacha (calamus root). It balances Vata, stabilizes moods, and improves clarity of thought.

AYURVEDIC THERAPIES
according to body type

	VATA	PITTA	KAPHA
GARSHANA	Balances	Balances	Balances
ABHYANGA	Balances	(Balances)	(Balances)
VISHESH	Aggravates	Neutral	Balances
UDVARTANA	Balances	(Aggravates)	Balances
SHIRODHARA	Balances	(Balances)	(Balances)
SWEDANA	Balances	Aggravates	Balances
FACIAL	Balances	Balances	Balances

Note: The effects of these treatments are described in detail in Chapter 5 and in Parts II and IV.

Chapter Five

Ayurvedic Massage Stroke Descriptions

Before I delve into the description of each massage stroke utilized in this manual, I want to reiterate the role of the therapist in Ayurvedic massage. When I was training in India, it was commonly mentioned that these therapies are better for the therapist than they are for the guest. As described in Chapter 2, the mindset of the therapist holds great importance for the success of the therapy. During an Ayurvedic massage the therapist has the opportunity to relearn how to think. Most of us in the West believe that in order to think we must think! But it is understood in Ayurveda that the faculty of thinking resides in the heart—under the auspices of feeling. So in fact to really learn to think we must learn to feel. Being able to function in life from this place of feeling, although not always accepted in the West, is a side benefit for an experienced Ayurvedic therapist. During the choreographed sequence of strokes, the mind of the therapist eventually lets go, and they begin to *feel* their way through the sequence rather than *think* their way through. In this non-thinking state the therapist and guest begin to communicate silently in a way that my teacher called soul to soul, or heart to heart.

From this feeling level of touch, the results can be profound. In Ayurveda the sense of touch used during massage relates to the element vayu. Vayu is like ayus, according to the *Sushruta Samhita:* "It is self-begotten in origin and is regarded as identical to eternal life or god itself." In the body this vayu is represented by the 10 pranas mentioned in Chapter 3. These pranas activate the 72,000 nadis, which in turn stimulate the six chakras that move the kundalini shakti up the spine to the thousand-petal lotus atop the head at the bindu point. This can happen only when awareness accompanies touch. The choreographed design of

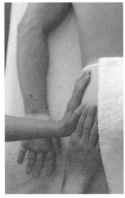

Whole Hand

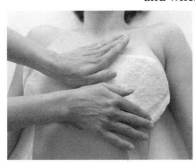

Palm

Ayurvedic massage ensures that the therapist does not get in the way of this subtle but profound process.

It is for this reason that all therapies are done in silence. The therapist instructs the guest to speak up only if the experience is uncomfortable in any way.

For the therapist there are some basic massage principles that will help to effect the desired result.

• **Whole hand.** Most strokes will use the whole hand—muscles of hand relaxed; hand soft and slightly cupped, and contoured to body.

• **Palm.** Central to abhyanga, the palm is the main source of contact. There are minor chakras on the palm of hand, and when the hand is opened these chakras are activated.

• **Thumb.** The thumb is adducted (held close to the index finger) except for Vishesh, where the thumb and index finger make a "V" for most strokes.

• **Fingers.** The fingers conform to the contour of the body area in a relaxed manner.

• **Pressure.** Pressure is balanced and even, using the whole hand as a unit, with even pressure on each finger and all four sides of the palm. Pressure is also body type specific:

> Vata types—lighter touch
> Pitta types—medium touch
> Kapha types—heavier touch

• **Strokes.** Strokes are long, full, and straight, making large circles around joints.

• **Touch.** Touch is with the whole hand and incorporates all the senses on a feeling level. During strokes the therapist must give full attention to the area being massaged. Touch gives rise to awareness, which gives rise to bliss.

Please note: The letters preceding stroke names throughout this chapter refer to the treatment(s) in which that stroke is used. **G**=Garshana, **A**=Abhyanga, **V**=Vishesh, **U**=Udvartana; **F**=Facial; a small **2** after the letter refers to the two-therapist modality. **ALL** means the stroke is used in every treatment. Most strokes are defined only for one-therapist treatments. Refer to two-therapist treatment chapters for variations.

In describing therapist positions, the right and left sides of the table are determined by the guest's right and left when lying supine.

It is difficult on a 2–dimensional photograph to indicate the direction of a stroke when its plane is at an angle to the viewer. For circular/oval strokes, the arrows point clockwise or counterclockwise to show the direction the therapist's hand moves on the body. Strokes on a body part that is not visible from the perspective of the photograph (e.g., on the back of the neck from a supine position) are indicated by dotted lines.

Head Massage

The head massage includes treatment of the face, scalp, head marmas, neck, and ears. Treatment of the head is always initiated while the guest is in a seated position. This is to engage the postural muscles of the spine in order to promote a state of self-awareness rather than a dull sleep state. Pranavaha and manovaha srotas and prana vayu channels are opened with the head massage. In addition, as the central nervous system controls the entire body, all srotas, vayus and nadis will be indirectly activated.

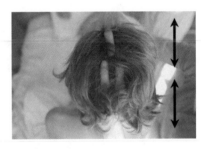

Head massage - top

Benefits of head massage: Nourishes the senses, relieves headaches, stops hair loss and premature graying, improves the complexion, and cures insomnia and Vata disorders.

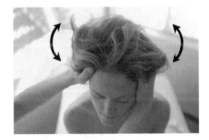

Head massage - sides

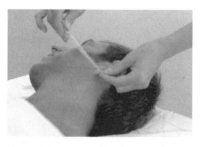

Karna Purana

AVU Karna Purana (supine): Pouring warm oil into the ears. **optional**

Benefits: Relieves earache, deafness, tinnitus, headache, lockjaw, torticollis (neck spasm), giddiness, tooth and gum problems; removes heat from the feet. It supports pranavaha, rasavaha, and manovaha srotas and balances prana and udana vayus. The nadis activated are: ida, pingala, shankhini, payasvati, gandhara, pusha, and susumna (see Chapter 3).

Caution: Karna purana is recommended only for guests doing a series of consecutive treatments, not just a day spa. As some people are more sensitive to oil being put in their ears, this part of the treatment is optional and up to the discretion of the therapist/guest.

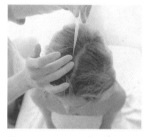

Simanta marma drops

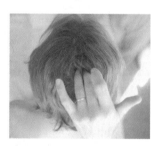

Adhipati marma massage

AVU Simanta Marma (seated): Coronal-parietal joint

AVU Adhipati Marma (seated): Back of head, occipital-parietal joint

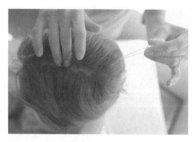

Simanta marma massage and adhipati marma drops

Marma therapy: Apply 10 drops of oil on simanta marma and rub gently in a clockwise circular motion about the size of a quarter—spiraling in for 5 seconds. Stop and gently hold this point while oil is dropped on the adhipati marma. Begin inward spirals on adhipati marma before taking the hand away from simanta marma.

Purpose: To establish self-awareness in the beginning of the treatment and to activate brain centers with each marma. This is done in the sitting position to avoid a sleep state and to increase awareness.

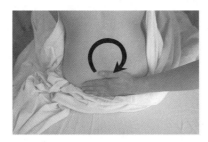

Seat of Vata circles - seated

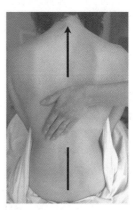

Sweep up spine

AVUF   Seat of Vata Circles (seated and prone): Quick clockwise circles on the small of the back (lumbosacral junction). After circles, sweep up the spine, neck, and off the head.

- Balances prana and apana vayus.
- Stimulates kundalini-carrying nadis in the base of the spine.
- Balances susumna, ida, and pingala with up-spine strokes.

AVU   Occipital Lift (seated): After the last set of Seat of Vata circles and up-spine stroke, with the index finger and thumb, lift and hold the occiput as the body is supported into a lying down position.

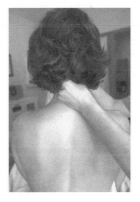

Benefits: Activates alertness established with head massage and marma treatment to enhance self-awareness as the body is put into a lying down position.

Hold at occiput

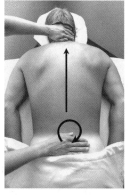

AVU Occipital Press (prone): After first hand Seat of Vata circles and sweep up spine, side of hand presses up against occiput while second hand does Seat of Vata circles and sweeps up spine. Then one hand follows other sweeping off head.

Seat of Vata circles and occipital press

Face Massage (all supine)

Benefits: Nourishes the senses, relieves tension, improves the complexion, helpful for Vata disorders.

Face Swipes: Using as much of a full hand as possible, start from chin (one hand on each side) and pull up sides of face, crossing hands to wrap around forehead.

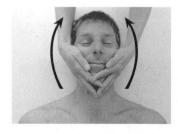
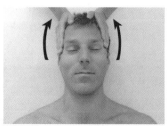
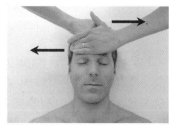

Face swipes - beginning   Face swipes - middle   Face swipes - end

Eyebrow Strokes: Stroke eyebrows with thumbs from nose to temples.

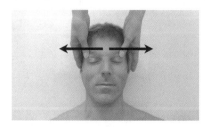

Eyebrow strokes

Eye Circles: With fingers, circle eyes starting from third eye, moving down bridge of nose, coming across under eyes, then back around to forehead.

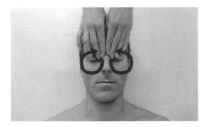

Eye circles

Bridge of Nose Stroke: With fingers, stroke down bridge and sides of nose, around outer nostrils and back up again.

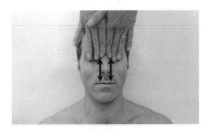

Bridge of nose strokes

Nostril Circles: Run fingertips around openings of nostrils.

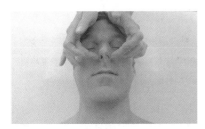

Nostril circles

Upper Lip Stroke: Using index finger, stroke above upper lip between lip line and nostrils.

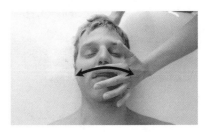

Upper lip strokes

Chin Bone Stroke: Using fingers of one hand, stroke back and forth across chin, along jaw bone.

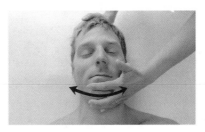

Chin bone strokes

Chin Circles: Alternating thumb circles on chin.

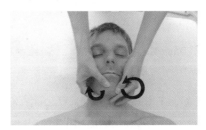

Chin circles

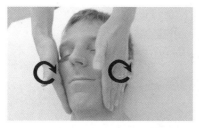

Cheek circles

Cheek Circles: Using hand (with soft fingers), make big, full circles coming up from chin, out along cheekbones and back down jaw line.

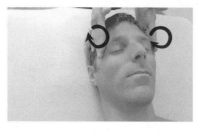

Temple circles

Temple Circles: Generous circles on temples with soft pads of fingers.

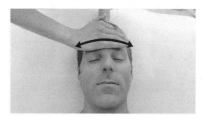

Forehead strokes

Forehead Stroke: With fingers soft and hand cupped, stroke palm back and forth across forehead, from temple to temple.

Ayurvedic Facial (uses all strokes in Face Massage section plus the following)

Full Back Circles: Starting at Seat of Vata, up paraspinals over scapulae, and down sides of body.

Reverse Full Back Circles: From neck, down paraspinals, up sides, hands meet again at neck; one hand follows other down and off Seat of Vata, then back up spine and off head.

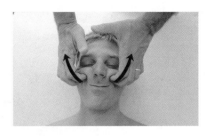

Maxilla Pulls: With fingers, hold maxilla bone and gently pull for 3–5 seconds (may travel slightly with each pull).

Maxilla pulls

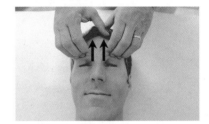

Eyebrow Pulls: With fingers, hold under the eyebrows and gently pull (may travel slightly with each pull).

Eyebrow pulls

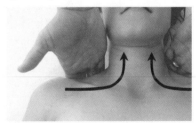

Trapezius to Occiput Strokes: Back and forth from shoulders to occiput.

Trapezius-to-occiput strokes

Ear Massage (supine)

Circles Up/Down: Pinching outer ear between thumb and index finger, work up ear with 10 circles, then down with 10.

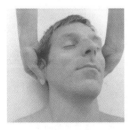

Circles up from bottom of ears

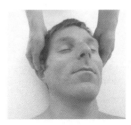

Circles down from top of ears

Scissors Strokes: With index and middle finger of both hands extended like scissors, stroke up and down sides of head with ears between fingers.

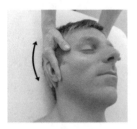

Neck Massage

Benefits: Neck strokes move udana vayu, which facilitates the flow of prana vayu into brain centers. In the same way, pranavaha and manovaha srotas are stimulated. Cervical lymph, or rasa, in the neck is massaged, activating the flow of rasavaha srotas. Nadis associated with the spine—ida, pingala, and susumna—are activated. Relieves congestion, tension, headaches, chronic colds, insomnia, and most Vata imbalances.

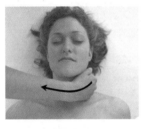

Horizontal neck swipes

AVU   Horizontal Neck Swipes (supine): Palm of hand and fingers alternately pull left and right across front of neck.

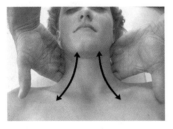

Cervical paraspinal strokes

GAVU   Cervical Paraspinal Strokes (supine/prone): Fingers are pressed along paraspinal muscles in an up-down motion.

ALL Trapezius Strokes
(supine/prone/side): Back and forth strokes from base of neck across upper trapezius muscles to shoulder. In side position, strokes go all the way from shoulder to occiput.

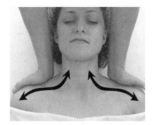

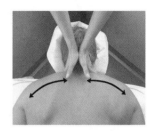

Trapezius strokes - prone

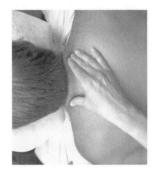

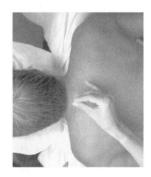

V Duck Bites (prone): Tips of thumb and fingers grab or "bite" back of neck and pull off multiple times, traveling from C7 to occiput.

Duck bite - beginning

Duck bite - end

VF Up/Down Neck Strokes (prone): With contoured hand cupped around spine, slide back and forth between C7 and occiput.

G Thyroid to Chin Alternating Neck Strokes (supine): With contoured hand, palm centered over thyroid, stroke is up neck to base of chin and off, alternating left and right hands.

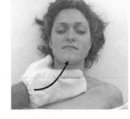

Thyroid to chin alternating neck strokes

A₂U Neck/Trap Strokes (side): Back and forth strokes between shoulder and occiput along upper traps.

A₂U Up Neck Sweep (side): Finishing stroke from shoulder up neck, behind ear, and off back of head.

Back Massage

The muscles of the back while supporting the limbs also hold up the spine and support the central nervous system. If these muscles are strained or tight, the srotas of the physical body will block any further subtle-body activation in the central nervous system. Consequently, after the head and feet, the back is next in importance.

The prana- and thought-carrying srotas (pranavaha, annavaha) are dependent upon a balanced back musculature. Vayus like apana and prana use the spine regularly through ida, pingala, and susumna nadis to maintain central nervous system function and to balance the subtle-body system. Circular strokes are for nadi activation, up-down spine strokes move vayus, and full coverage strokes move srotas.

AUF Scapula Circles (prone/side): With full hand, down scapula strokes move down center of spine and up around scapula. Up scapula strokes go up spine and down around scapula. Both strokes end at heart.

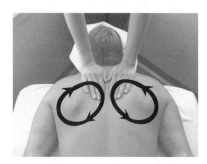

Scapula circles - down

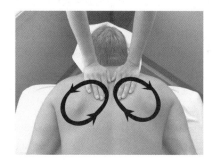

Scapula circles - up

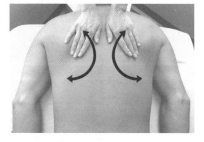

Crescent moon strokes

AUF Crescent Moon Strokes (prone/side): From head of table, strokes are in shape of crescent across superior, medial, and inferior borders of scapula to side of body and back.

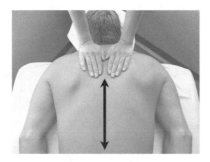

Paraspinal strokes - beginning

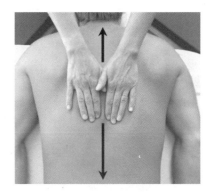

Paraspinal strokes -middle

AVUF Paraspinal Strokes (prone/side): With one hand on each side of spine, stroke up and/or down paraspinal muscles with full hand.

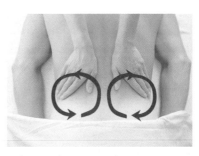

AUF Kidney Circles (prone): Up kidney circles come up center of back and down sides. Circles are grapefruit size and slightly faster paced than rest of back strokes. Down kidney circles go down midline then up sides. Use lighter pressure over kidneys.

Kidney circles - up

AU One-Handed Traveling Up/Down Circles Across Kidneys (side): Side-position version of kidney circles; both kidneys done with one hand. Circles are same but moving back and forth from one kidney to other, traveling in clockwise circles up from the table and counterclockwise back down again.

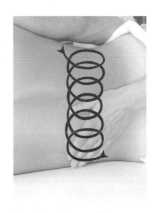

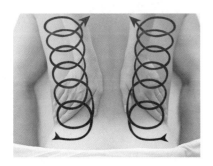

AUF Back Spirals (prone/side): Eight overlapping circles that move from Seat of Vata up back and end wrapped over top of shoulders.

One-handed traveling up/down kidney circles

Back spirals

AU   Full Coverage Back Strokes (prone): Using full hands, strokes go down paraspinal muscles, across iliac crest, then pull up sides.

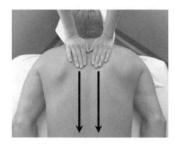 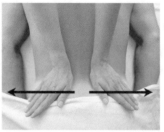 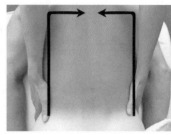

Full coverage back strokes -
beginning

Full coverage back strokes -
middle

Full coverage back strokes - end

A_2U_2 One-Handed Full Coverage Back Strokes (prone): Same as full coverage back strokes, but staying on one side of spine.

GAU   Crisscross Back Strokes (prone/side): From side of table, starting at Seat of Vata, hands slide in opposite directions, crisscrossing spine, going up to shoulder and back down to starting point (refer to variations in individual treatments).

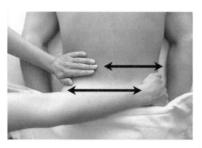 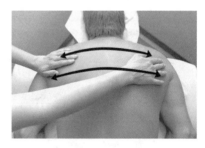

Crisscross strokes - at sacrum

Crisscross strokes - at shoulder

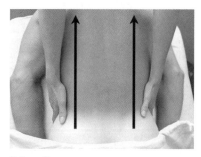

Side pulls

VUF Side Pulls (prone): From head of table hands wrap around sides of body just above hip with fingers barely touching table and pull up to axilla.

U$_2$ One-Handed Side Pulls (prone): Same as side pulls, but on only one side of body.

V$_2$ Up Side Strokes (prone): Starting at hips, facing head of table, one hand on each side slides up axillary line.

V Pivoting Half Moons (prone): Down stroke—starting facing guest's head, thumbs interlocked, fingers wrapped over shoulder and barely touching table, therapist pivots to face guest's feet while firmly sliding hands in arc over scapula. Lift off, pivot back to starting position and repeat. Up stroke—reverse starting and ending positions.

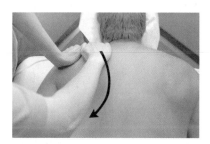

Pivoting half moon - down

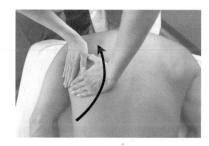

Pivoting half moon - up

V Paraspinal Finger Strokes (prone): With fingers sliding along paraspinal muscles, strokes are up or down with firm pressure, going from seat of Vata to top of shoulders.

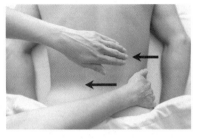

Alternating pulls

V Alternating Pulls (prone): From side of table, reaching across to opposite side of body, left and right hands alternate pulling from side across to spine and lifting off, working their way from hip to top of shoulder and back down to hip.

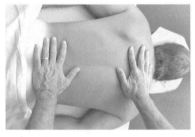

Gentle rocking and smoothing

V Rocking and Smoothing (prone): Using firm pressure, gently rock the body for 5–10 seconds.

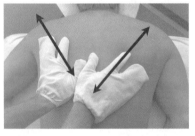

Garshana - "V" strokes

G "V" Strokes: From side of table, starting from mid-back, strokes go back and forth in shape of "V" moving up and out to top of shoulders and back to heart.

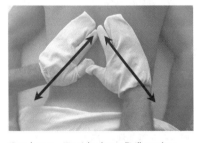

Garshana - Upside down "V" strokes

G Upside-Down "V" Strokes: From side of table, starting from mid-back, strokes move back and forth in shape of upside-down "V" following rib line down and out to top of hips, then back to heart.

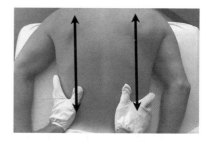

G **Up/Down Side Strokes:** From side of table, hands slide briskly up and down axillary line from hips to lower edge of scapula.

Garshana - Up/down side strokes

Hello/Goodbye Sweeps

Sweeps typically begin and end every therapy as well as each section of the therapy. These strokes merge the circulation of one body part with another, with the goal of integrating them as one. Sweeps are very powerful therapeutically and feel wonderful to the guest. As sweeps encompass the whole body, they activate all the srotas, vayus, and nadis. Sweeps are slow with medium pressure.

(Refer to each treatment for variation details.)

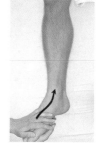

AVU Hello Sweep (supine/prone): Giving as much coverage to contours of body as possible, stroke moves from toes up leg, up torso, around shoulder and down arm—then back up arm, transitioning to next body part (supine = cervical spine, prone = Seat of Vata).

Sweep - foot

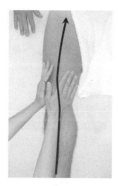
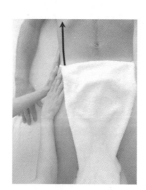
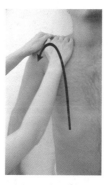
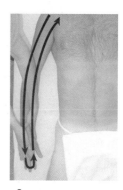

Sweep - leg   Sweep - torso   Sweep - shoulder   Sweep - arm

A₂U Hello Leg Sweep (side): Starting at hip, sweep down leg to toes and back up to hip again.

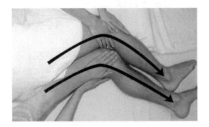
Sweep down leg - 2 therapists

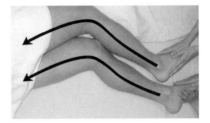
Sweep up leg - 2 therapists

AVU Goodbye Arm Sweep (supine/prone): Moves from fingers to shoulder, down torso or back, down leg, and off foot.

AVU Goodbye Leg Sweep (supine/prone): Moves from toes, up leg to hip, back down to toes and is usually followed by goodbye full-body sweep.

AVU Goodbye Full Body Sweep (supine/prone): Moves from toes, up leg, up torso/back to shoulder, down arm to fingers, back up arm to shoulder, down back/torso, leg, and off foot.

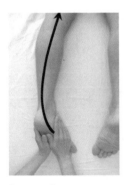
Sweep - foot

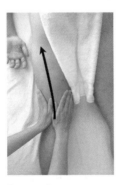
Sweep - leg

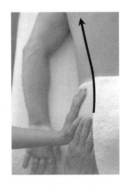
Sweep - hip/back

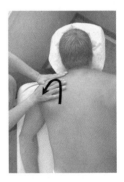
Sweep - shoulder

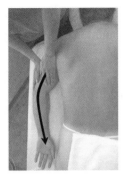
Sweep - down arm

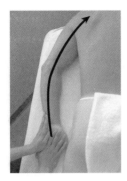
Sweep - up arm

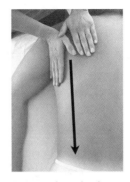
Sweep - down back

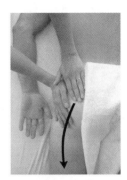
Sweep - down leg

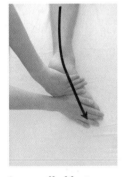
Sweep off of foot

$A_2V_2U_2$ · **Finishing Sweeps for Feet** (supine): Doing both feet at once, starting at toes, sweep up along front of legs to about mid-calf, fan hands out to wrap around calves, sweep back down to toes. Repeat two more times. End by coming off foot, twisting in to get arch and pulling off toes.

Foot Massage

Next to the head, the foot is the most important area of the body to massage. The foot is well nourished with blood supply and capillary beds and has a concentration of nerve endings. According to Vagbhata (author of the Ayurvedic text *Astanga-hridaya*) there are four major nerves in the soles of the feet that are connected to the eyes. Because of the friction, excessive pressure, and heat caused by walking, these nerves become afflicted and eyesight gets distorted. Ayurvedic strokes on the feet also support the function of the ears and help to relieve sciatica; insomnia; fatigue; cramps; and contraction of ligaments, vessels, and muscles of the lower limbs.

Because of the concentrated blood vessels in the feet, massage affects all seven of the deep tissues, thus activating rasavaha, raktavaha, mamsavaha, medavaha, asthivaha, majjavaha, and shukravaha srotas. Svedavaha srotas, which carry sweat, are also abundant in the feet. Apana vayu—or the downward flowing vayu—is stimulated, activating hastijihva and yashasvati nadis (that regulate the limbs) and gandhari and pusha nadis (that control sight, which is directly connected to the soles of the feet).

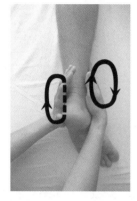 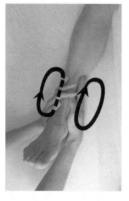

GAU   Bicycle Ankle Circles (supine/prone): Full handed, fast alternating circles around medial and lateral malleoli.

Bicycle ankle circles - prone   Bicycle ankle circles - supine

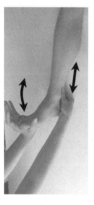

AVU   Achilles Tendon Strokes (supine/prone): Thumb and index finger of inside hand strip Achilles tendon from calcaneus to gastrocnemius bifurcation while outside hand flexes and extends ankle joint by applying pressure at toes.

Achilles tendon strokes

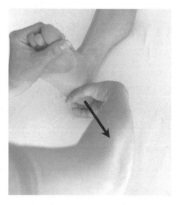

AVU   Thumb/Heel Strokes (supine): Grab heel with side of thumb at mid-sole, squeezing thumb along plantar fascia off the calcaneus with firm pressure.

Thumb/heel strokes

AU Shoeshine Strokes (supine/prone): One hand supports foot while other hand rapidly strokes up and down dorsal surface from ankle to toes.

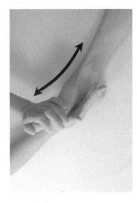

Shoeshine strokes

AU Alternating Squeezes (supine): Hands grab sides of foot with fingers wrapped around to mid-sole. Alternate left and right pulls and squeezes off the foot.

ALL Milk Toes (supine/prone): From foot of table, thumbs on top of foot, fingers holding bottom of foot, pull thumbs between metatarsals, sliding thumbs between toes, squeezing and pulling off toes. Work from sides to middle of foot, finishing with pull off middle toe.

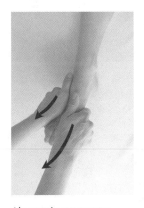

Alternating squeezes

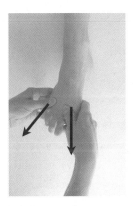

Milk toes - supine beginning

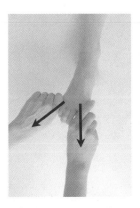

Milk toes - supine pulling off toes

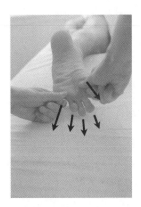

Milk toes - prone pulling off toes

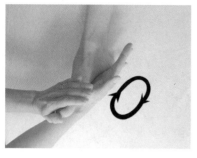

Ovals

AU   Ovals (supine/prone): Full hand does fast ovals around entire plantar surface of foot.

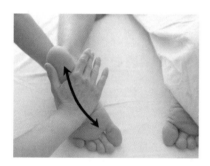

Full arch strokes - prone

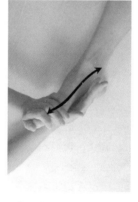

Full arch strokes - supine

AU   Full Arch Strokes (supine/prone): With full palm, stroke is up and down over arch from base of heel to base of toes.

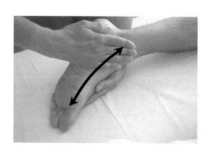

Inside arch strokes - prone

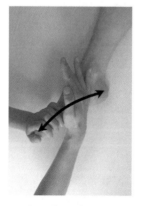

Inside arch strokes - supine

AU   Inside Arch Strokes (supine/prone): Using outside edge and palm of hand, stroke up and down over medial edge of arch.

AU   Outside Arch Strokes
(supine/prone): Using same
hand as inside arch strokes,
stroke lateral edge of arch with
index edge and palm of hand.

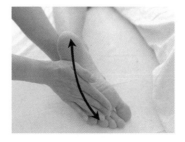

Outside arch strokes - prone

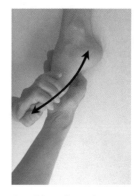

Outside arch strokes -
supine

**GAU   Combo Shoeshine/Oval
Strokes** (supine/prone): While
one hand is making ovals on
sole of foot, other is doing
shoeshine strokes on top of
foot.

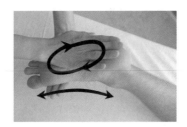

Combo shoeshine/oval strokes -
prone

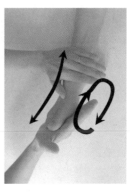

Combo shoeshine/oval
strokes - supine

V   Heel Squeeze (prone): From mid-sole, with pressure from oppos-
ing index and thumb, slide up sides of heel, squeezing off back of
heel.

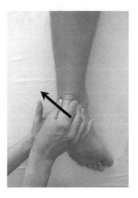

Heel squeezes

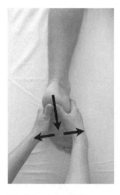
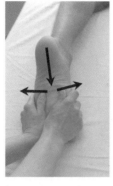

AVU Upside-Down "T" Press (prone): On sole of foot, thumbs slide with firm pressure from base of heel to base of toes, then spread like upside-down T.

Upside-down "T" press - beginning

Upside-down "T" press - end

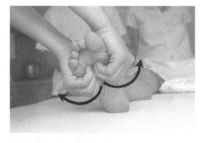

AVU Metatarsal Spread (supine): Hands grab sides of foot. As thumbs press and spread metatarsals, fingers press into plantar surface of foot and pull outward.

Metatarsal spread

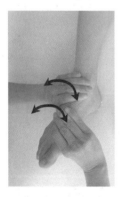

A_2VU_2 **Wringing Strokes** (supine): Grabbing foot with thumbs hooked underneath pressing on sole, fingers overlap on top of foot and with wringing motion massage top and sides of foot.

Wringing strokes

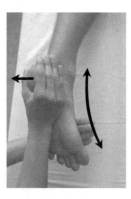

AU Heel Squeezes/Shoeshine Strokes (prone): Combine heel squeeze and shoeshine strokes.

Combo heel
squeezes/shoeshine strokes

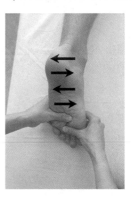

V Thumb Crisscross (prone): Stroke back and forth with thumbs up sole of foot from toes to heel.

Thumbs crisscross up
bottom of feet

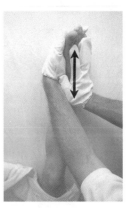

G Toe Web Strokes (supine/prone): With therapist's fingers pointing in same direction as guest's toes and fitted between toes on dorsal side of foot, massage inner webs of all toes simultaneously.

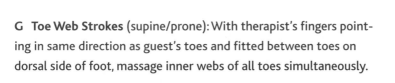

Garshana - Toe web strokes

Hand Massage

Like the foot, the hand has a concentration of nerves and blood supply. However, it does not have the same impact on the central nervous or subtle-body systems as the foot. Massaging a distal extremity activates lymph channels or rasavaha srotas, which, being the first and most common srotas, will in turn activate the others. Distal circulation is regulated by vyana vayu and samana vayu, which control lymph movement. Activating minor chakras on the palms of the hand activates the nadi system.

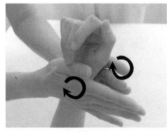

Bicycle wrist circles

Note: for the first three strokes, the arm is flexed at the elbow.

GAU   Bicycle Wrist Circles (supine): Fast, small, alternating circles on anterior and posterior sides of wrist.

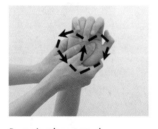

Pumping heart strokes

AU   Pumping Heart Strokes (supine): Holding hand with thumbs on palm, knead around palm in shape of heart.

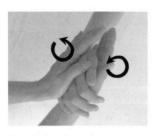

Bicycle hand circles

GAU   Bicycle Hand Circles (supine): Fast, alternating circles on anterior and posterior sides of hand (metacarpals).

ALL   Milk Fingers (supine/prone): From side of table, thumbs on top of hand, fingers on bottom, pull thumbs between metacarpals, squeeze along length of fingers and pull off fingertips. Work from sides to middle of hand, finishing with pull off middle finger.

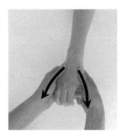
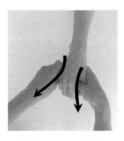
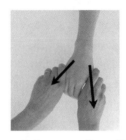
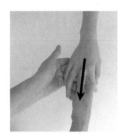

Milk fingers - metacarpals

Milk fingers - web of fingers

Milk fingers - pulling off fingers

Milk fingers - pulling off middle finger

AU   Alternating Squeezes (supine): Hands grab sides of guest's hand with fingers wrapped around to palm. Alternate left and right pulls and squeezes off the hand.

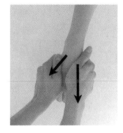

Alternating squeezes

G   Finger Web Strokes (supine/prone): With therapist's fingers pointing same directions as and fitting between guest's fingers on dorsal side of hand, massage inner webs of all fingers simultaneously.

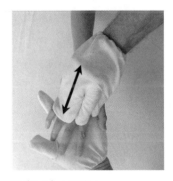

Right side position

Torso Massage (all supine)

The chest and abdomen are the most vulnerable parts of the body. It is from the front of the body that the vital organs are most accessible and are nourished. Thus all the nourishing srotas are primarily activated, like annavaha srotas that carry food, the seven dhatu srotas, and pranavaha and ambhuvaha srotas that carry energy and water. Lighter pressure should be used over the heart and gastrointestinal areas.

Samana and apana vayus have their seats on the torso and regulate digestion, assimilation, and elimination. As a consequence, there are many nadis activated, which results in chakra stimulation. Circular strokes improve nadi and chakra function, while whole torso strokes move the srotas and vayus.

AU Pectoral Circles: Both up and down strokes begin over the heart. Down pectoral strokes move down the sternum and around the breast to the axilla and back to the heart. Up pectoral strokes go around the breast and up the sternum. For women the stroke goes around the breast, activating more axilla and lymph drainage. For men the stroke goes over the breast.

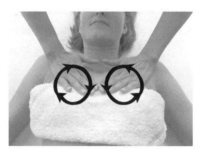
Pectoral circles - down

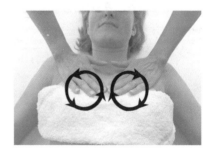
Pectoral circles - up

V Two-Handed Pectoral Circles: With one hand on top of other, perform movements as described for pectoral circles.

AV Side Squares: From head of table (side for a two-therapist treatment) stroke goes down mammillary line just below breast to just above hip level, moves posterior, and then pulls back up the posterior lateral portion of the rib cage.

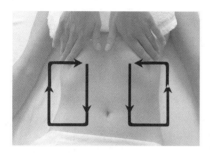
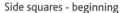

Side squares - beginning

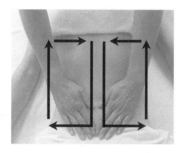

Side squares - middle

A Whole Torso Circles: From head of table, full hands move down the midline (sternum), pull up sides (around breast for women, over breast for men) and then down midline again.

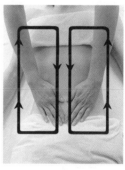

Whole torso circles

U Whole Torso Circles: Beginning with heels of hands just above hip joint with fingers pointed toward midline, pull out to side, shift position of hands so fingers point down, continue up sides of body to axilla, then follow through to heart. Move hands down midline, returning to starting position to begin next circle.

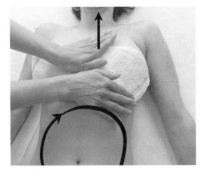

Heart/stomach strokes

AU Heart/Stomach Strokes: From right side of table, left hand is slowly stroking along sternum, over heart, while right hand is doing large, slow, clockwise abdominal circles. This is an unhurried, calming stroke. Both hands should meet at xiphoid process after each circle/stroke and pause after final stroke.

GAVU Butterfly Stroke: With thumbs interlocked and hands in shape of butterfly, starting at guest's side just above hip, stroke goes up to shoulder for men, ends just below breast for women. Stroke is also used during sweeps and may be continued to shoulder. Sweeps may use butterfly strokes in supine or prone.

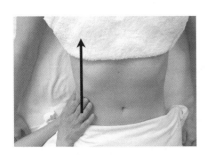

Butterfly stroke

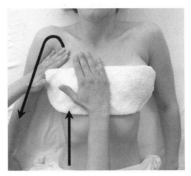

Butterfly stroke transitioning to sweep

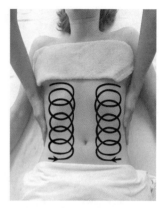

Up side spirals

U Up Side Spirals: From head of table reaching down to guest's sides just above hips (hands wrapped around small of back, fingers barely touching table) work up sides to axilla (below breast for women) with small spirals.

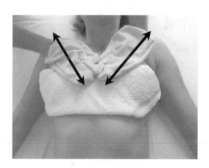

"V" strokes

G "V" Strokes: From side of table, starting from sternum, strokes go back and forth in shape of "V" moving up and out to each shoulder and back to heart.

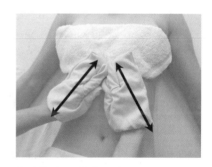

Upside-down "V" strokes

G Upside-Down "V" Strokes: From side of table, starting from sternum, strokes move back and forth in shape of upside-down "V" following rib line down and out to sides, then back to heart.

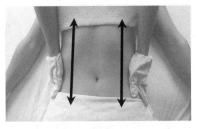

Up/down side strokes

G Up/Down Side Strokes: From side or head of table, hands move briskly up and down axillary line from hips to breast level.

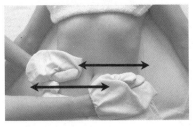

Crisscross stomach strokes

G Crisscross Stomach Strokes: From side of table, hands move in opposite directions, crisscrossing over abdomen from below navel to xiphoid process.

Limb Massage

According to Ayurveda, the limbs connect the concentrated nerve plexuses and capillary beds on the hands and feet to the circulation center and central nervous system in the torso. At the major junction points (shoulders, hips, knees, elbows, ankles, and wrists), powerful marma points and minor chakras and nadi plexuses exist, which is why these joints are treated with special attention. All joints receive circular motions with as much full hand coverage as possible, which brings awareness to the points and stimulates blood flow, vayu activity, and enhanced self-awareness through marma point activation. In addition, the circular strokes are directed at stimulating the nadis and the minor chakras (which spin) within each of the main joints.

Up/down strokes on the long bones are like the railroad tracks between stations (the stations being the joints). These strokes support circulation, but treat the subtle-body system as well.

Throughout the leg and arm sections, you will find references to "planes." In the supine position, both the arm and leg have three planes:

outside (lateral), top, and inside (medial). In the prone position, the leg still has three planes, but the arm has only one.

In the side-lying position, both arm and leg have two planes, inside and outside. To visualize these planes for the legs, imagine the guest is wearing a snugly fitting pair of pants. When the therapist's *fingers* ride along the seam, their hand is working the *inside* plane. When the therapist's *palm* rides along the seam, their hand is working the *outside* plane.

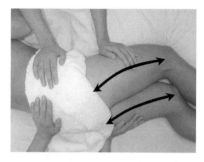

Upper leg strokes on inside plane

You can similarly visualize the planes of the arm by imagining where the crease in the guest's shirt sleeve would fall.

GAVU Circles at Joints—shoulder, elbow, wrist, hip, buttock, knee, ankle (supine/prone): Full handed with as much palm as possible, circles are performed on the appropriate plane indicated.

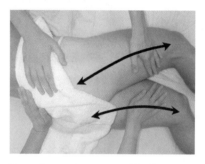

Upper leg strokes on outside plane

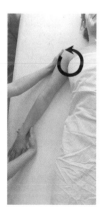

Shoulder circles - outside plane

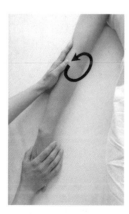

Elbow circles - outside plane

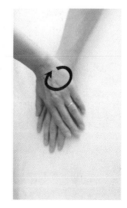

Wrist circles - top plane

Note that for top plane buttock circles, pressure has posterior to anterior emphasis (not medial to lateral), taking care not to spread gluteal crease.

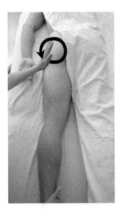

Hip circles - outside plane

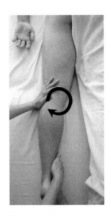

Knee circles - top plane

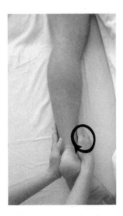

Ankle circles - inside plane

GAVU   Strokes at Long Bones—calf, upper leg, forearm, upper arm (supine/prone): With full hand, strokes are back and forth from joint to joint on indicated plane. It is crucial to overlap joints at each end of long bone.

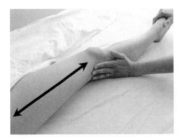

Long bone strokes - outside plane of upper leg

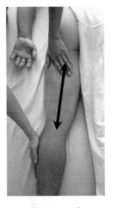

Long bone strokes - top plane

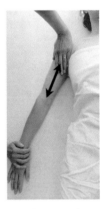

Long bone strokes - top plane of upper arm

V Alternating "V" Pushes (supine/prone): Using web in "V" between thumb and index finger, alternate strokes with right and left hand, stripping musculature in a firm motion pushing distally along arms/legs.

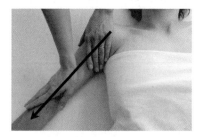

Alternating "V" pushes - upper arm

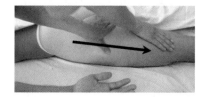

Alternating "V" pushes - upper leg

V Wringing Strokes (supine/prone): With two hands firmly holding arm or leg, limb is wrung out with back and forth motion working distally. For arm, wringing goes from shoulder to wrist, ending with squeeze off hand. For leg in supine, wring from hip to toes, then squeeze off foot from ankle to toes. In prone, wring from hip to ankle, then press off foot.

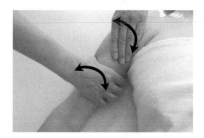

Wringing strokes on arm

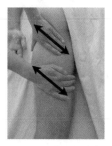

Wringing strokes on thigh

V Calf Wrap-Around (supine): Knee bent, cover foot with washcloth or sheet, therapist sits on toes. Inside hand holds knee, outside hand starts at inside of ankle, pulls up medially, down laterally 10 times. Switch so outside hand holds knee, inside hand starts at outside of ankle, pulls up laterally, down medially 10 times, ending down.

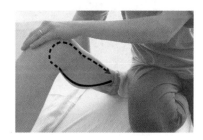

Calf wrap-around

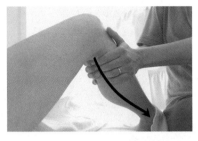

Calf squeezes

V Calf Squeezes (supine): With knee bent and therapist sitting on toes, calf muscle is squeezed with both hands simultaneously, pulling downward from knee to just above ankle.

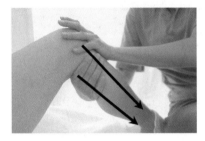

Calf press-off

V Calf Press-Off (supine): Starting with one hand covering kneecap and other behind knee, make one long, squeezing pull down to ankle and off top of foot.

V Pivoting Half Moons (prone): Down stroke—starting facing guest's head, thumbs interlocked, fingers wrapped over iliac crest, outside hand barely touching table, therapist pivots to face guest's feet while firmly sliding hands in arc over buttock. Lift off, pivot back to starting position and repeat. Up stroke—reverse starting and ending positions.

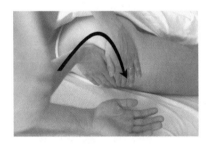
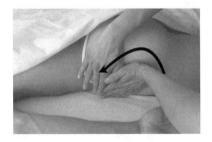

Pivoting half moon on buttocks

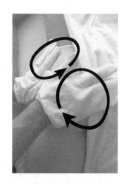

G   Polishing Circles (prone): Alternating right and left hand circles covering entire surface of buttock, following contours.

Garshana - Outward polishing circles

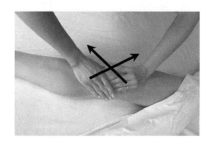

V   Kneecap Squeezes (supine): With index fingers and thumbs, kneecap is kneaded from above and below, alternating left and right hand squeezes, toward center of knee and off.

Kneecap squeezes

Shirodhara (all supine)

Horizontal Pattern: Directing dhara (oil stream) across forehead, starting just above eyebrows, going from ear to ear without losing oil contact, working up to just past hairline.

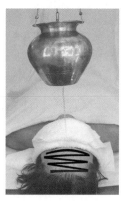

Shirodhara - Horizontal (Pitta)

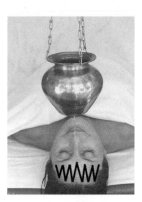

Vertical Pattern: Like a zigzag/up-down pattern working back and forth across forehead.

Shirodhara - Vertical (Kapha)

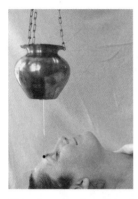

Shirodhara - 3rd eye (Vata)

Stationary Pattern: Holding oil stream over third eye for extended period of time.

PART II

One-Person Massage Therapies

While Ayurvedic massage is classically done with two therapists, one-person Ayurvedic massage therapies are also highly effective. The therapies described in this section are the classic Ayurvedic treatments performed by an Ayurvedic massage therapist. Each treatment has a unique and specific effect on the physical- and subtle-body systems. It is important that an Ayurvedic massage therapist understand the effects of each of these treatments in order to maximize therapeutic results.

Each of these therapies is precisely choreographed and leaves very little individual creativity for the massage therapist. At first this may seem limiting, however once the dance is committed to memory, the mind transcends the massage, allowing therapist and client to slip into a heart to heart or soul to soul communion. The massage therapist is not the "healer," but one who enhances the experience of self-awareness for the client, thus supporting a natural and spontaneous healing process.

Chapter Six

Garshana

The word garshana means "rubbing." There are actually two types of garshana:

- Internal garshana—during physical exercise.
- External garshana—vigorous body massage with wool, raw silk, or cotton.[1]

Garshana is a form of exfoliation that can occur both internally and externally. Exercise increases circulation and stimulates the flow of nourishing and waste-removing srotas as a form of internal garshana. Vigorously massaging the body with wool, raw silk, or terry cloth creates an external effect of increasing heat in the skin. Heat improves circulation, which stimulates the srotas to remove waste and nourish the body. In fact, all sixteen srotas are stimulated.

External garshana also increases static electricity in and around the body, an important part of the therapy.[1] Static electricity has been understood as a powerful healing modality in Ayurvedic medicine. In the 1900s scientists used a variety of devices and brushes to create static electricity and administer this current to patients. The effect creates an ionization and alkalization of the blood. The static electricity increases heat, and of course channels of circulation and waste removal are improved. Similarly, the wool or silk gloves, which are most commonly used, produce a static electricity charge that is directed back into the patient during the garshana massage. Conditions that benefit from static electricity massage, according to the Ministry of Health and Welfare in Japan, include:

- Headache
- Stiffness and muscle aches

- Neuralgia
- Fatigue
- Blood circulation
- Gastrointestinal function

Garshana massage is orchestrated much like udvartana where most of the strokes are in an upward direction that helps stimulate lymphatic flow. This particularly activates lymph-moving srotas like rasavaha srotas.

The exfoliating effect of garshana is measurable as the raw silk and wool are fairly abrasive yet soothing to the skin. Once the skin is exfoliated it functions better, especially as a large organ to eliminate waste.

The improved circulation of the sixteen srotas helps to initiate the flow of the vayus, which in turn initiates the activation of the nadis. The static electricity has a beneficial effect on the nadis and chakras because they function within the electromagnetic field.

Garshana is typically done before Ayurvedic massage or before bathing. It is recommended to be done daily and can be for any body type. Raw silk gloves are for Vata and Pitta types and wool for Kapha. Terry cloth is also used sometimes for Vata and Pitta types.

1.   Venimadhashastri Joshi, Lecture excerpt (Fairfield, IA, Nov. 10, 1986). Resides: Bombay, India.

One-Therapist Garshana
2 positions
10–15 minutes

Purpose

Garshana is a dry massage done with wool, raw silk, or terry cloth gloves. This massage is performed quickly over the skin and removes dead skin cells, stimulating the circulation and the lymphatic system. This massage can be done before any body treatment.

Massage Technique

Garshana is performed using wool, raw silk, or terry cloth gloves (depending on guest's body type). Both hands move together in synchrony.

For multiple days of treatment, long bone strokes can increase by increments of 10 each day. Maximum count is 60 strokes per area.

Two-Position Garshana—One Therapist

Position 1

Guest Position: Lying supine with towel covering body. Support knees and neck as needed. Fold towel or sheet appropriately. No oil is applied to body.

Therapist Position: Start at feet, facing head.

• Hello full-body sweep

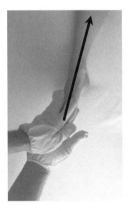
Sweep up foot

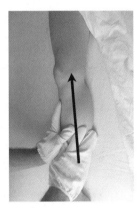
Sweep up calf

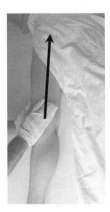
Sweep up thigh

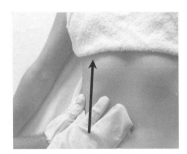
Sweep up torso

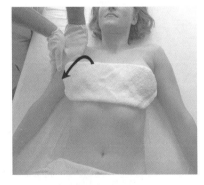
Sweep down shoulder

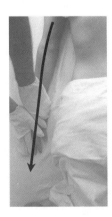
Sweep down arm to hand

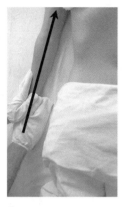

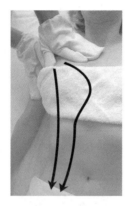

Sweep up arm to shoulder

Sweep down torso

Foot

- Milk toes
- 10 toe web strokes
- 10 combo shoeshine/oval strokes
- Come off foot

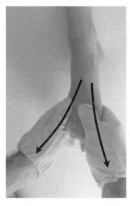

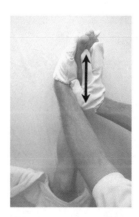

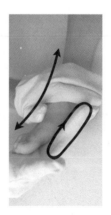

Milk toes

Toe web strokes

Combo shoeshine/oval strokes

Leg (Hands cover all three planes simultaneously. Strokes are up and down, with hands moving in synchrony.)

Therapist Position: Foot of table, facing guest's head. Start with right foot.

- 5 bicycle ankle circles
- 20 calf strokes

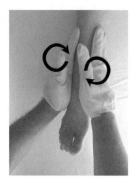

Bicycle ankle circles

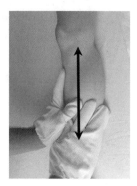

Calf strokes

Therapist Position: Right side of table.

- 5 knee circles
- 20 upper leg strokes
- 5 one-handed hip circles
- 5 up/down butterfly strokes
- Follow through down to hand

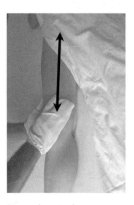

Upper leg strokes

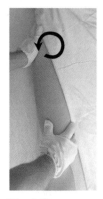

Hip circles

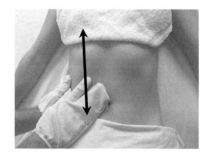

Butterfly stroke

Hand

- Milk Fingers

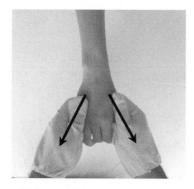

Milk fingers - beginning

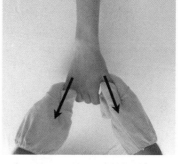

Milk fingers - pulling off of fingers

- 10 finger web strokes
- 10 bicycle hand circles
- Come off hand

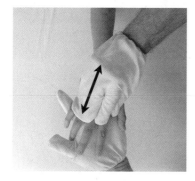

Finger web strokes

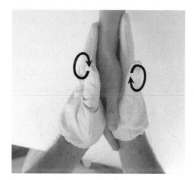

Bicycle hand circles

Arm (Hands cover all three planes simultaneously. Strokes are up and down, with hands moving in synchrony.)

Therapist Position: Right side of table, facing guest's head.

- 5 bicycle wrist circles
- 20 forearm strokes
- 5 elbow circles
- 20 upper arm strokes

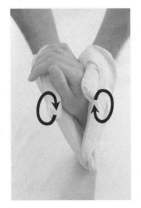 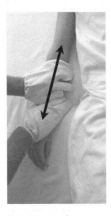 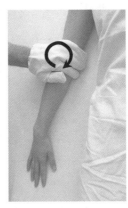 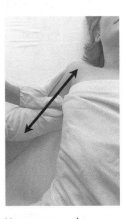

Bicycle wrist circles   Forearm strokes   Elbow circles   Upper arm strokes

- 5 two-handed shoulder circles
- Sweep down to hand
- Goodbye arm sweep

Therapist Position: Move to left side of table. Repeat entire leg and arm sequence from left side of table, beginning with hello full-body sweep. On goodbye arm sweep, do not go back down leg. Stay at torso.

Torso

Therapist Position: Left side of table, facing guest.

- 10 "V" strokes
- 10 upside-down "V" strokes

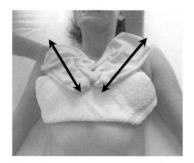

"V" strokes

Upside-down "V" strokes

- 10 up/down side strokes
- 10–20 alternating crisscross stomach strokes

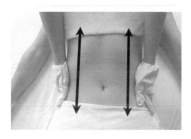
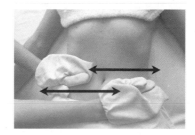

Up/down side strokes

Crisscross stomach strokes

Therapist Position: Move to head of table.

Neck

- 5 up/down cervical paraspinal strokes

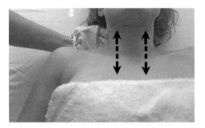

Traps

- 5 up/down trapezius strokes

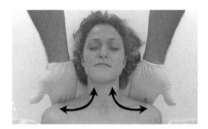

Face

- 3 face swipes

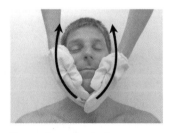

Face swipes - beginning

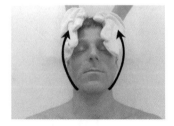

Face swipes - middle

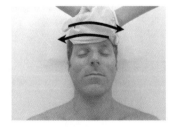

Face swipes - end

- 5 eyebrow strokes
- 5 eye circles
- 5 bridge of nose strokes
- 5 nostril circles
- 5 upper lip strokes

- 5 chin bone strokes
- 5 chin circles
- 5 cheek circles
- 5 temple circles
- 5 forehead strokes

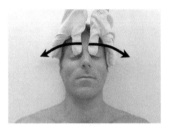

Eyebrow strokes

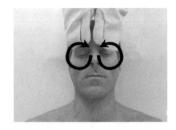

Eye circles

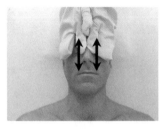

Bridge of nose strokes

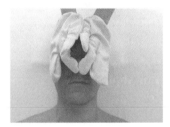

Nostril circles

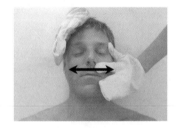

Upper lip strokes

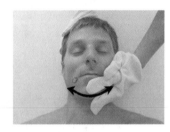

Chin bone strokes

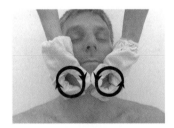

Chin circles

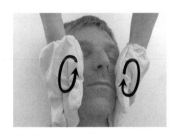

Cheek circles

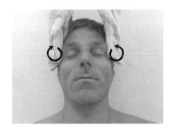

Temple circles

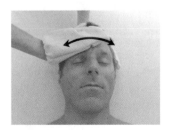

Forehead strokes

Ears

- 10 circles up
- 10 circles down

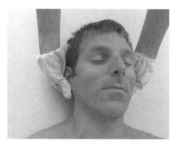

- 10 scissors strokes

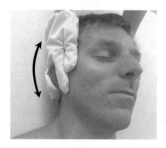

Neck

- 10 thyroid to chin alternating neck strokes

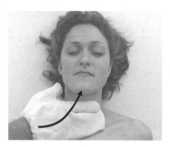

Face

- 3 face swipes (on last swipe, both hands come off top of head)

Two-Position Garshana—One Therapist

Position 2

Guest Position: Lying prone.

Therapist Position: Move to right side of table. Instruct guest to lie prone. Offer face cradle. Drape appropriately. If needed, place pillow under ankles.

- Hello full-body sweep

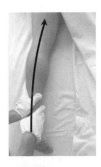
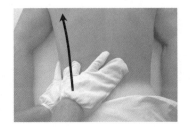
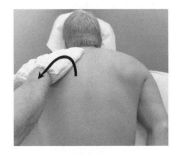

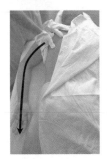
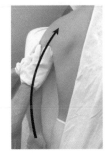
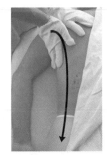
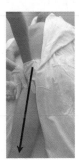

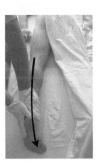

Foot
- 10 toe web strokes
- 10 combo shoeshine/oval strokes
- Come off foot

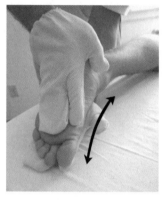
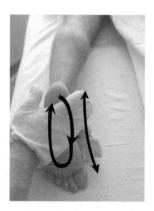
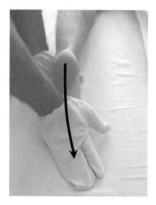

Toe web strokes   Combo shoeshine/oval strokes   Come off foot

Leg (Hands cover all three planes simultaneously. Strokes are up and down, with hands moving in synchrony.)

Therapist Position: Foot of table, facing guest's head. Start at left foot.

- 5 bicycle ankle circles
- 20 calf strokes

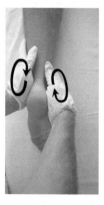
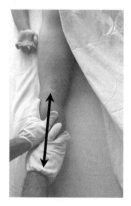

Bicycle ankle circles   Calf strokes

Therapist Position: Right side of table.
- 5 knee circles
- 20 upper leg strokes
- 5 hip circles

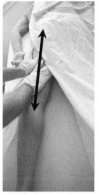 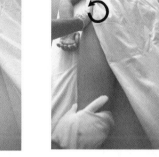

Upper leg strokes   Hip circles

Buttock

- 10 polishing circles

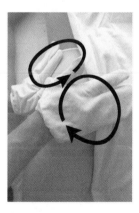

Back

- 10 up/down butterfly strokes

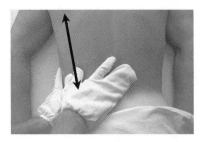

- Follow through down to hand

Arm

Therapist Position: Right side of table, facing guest's head.

- 10 finger web strokes
- 5 one-handed wrist circles
- 20 forearm strokes

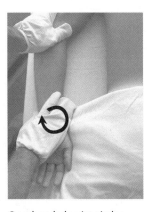 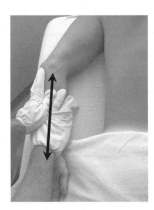

One-handed wrist circles   Forearm strokes

- 5 elbow circles
- 20 upper arm strokes
- 5 outside shoulder circles

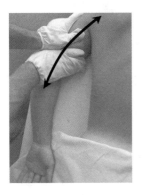
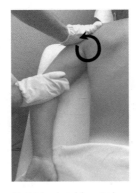

Upper arm strokes   Outside shoulder circles

- Sweep down arm
- Goodbye arm sweep

Therapist Position: Move to left side of table. Repeat entire leg and arm sequence from left side of table, beginning with hello full-body sweep.

On goodbye arm sweep, do not go back down the leg. Stay at back.

Back

Therapist Position: Left side of table, facing guest's head.

- 10 "V" strokes
- 10 upside-down "V" strokes

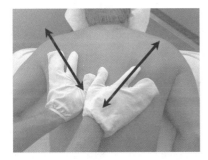
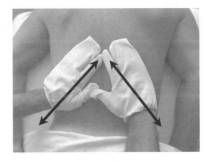

"V" strokes   Upside-down "V" strokes

- 10 up/down side strokes
- Crisscross back strokes up/down/up back, then both hands come off head

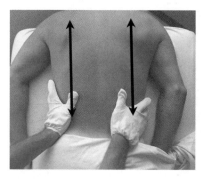 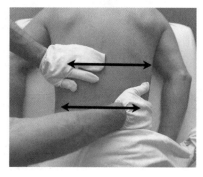

Up/down side strokes   Crisscross strokes

Chapter Seven

Abhyanga

In Sanskirt, *abhy* = to rub and *anga* = limb, so together they form the word for massage. Abhyanga is considered the classic Ayurvedic massage technique to prepare the body for panchakarma. Primarily it is a technique used to oleate or unctuate—that is, to impregnate the body with herbalized oils through massage. There are many variations of an Ayurvedic abhyanga, all basically derived from the same source with similar goals. As discussed in Chapter 3, the goal is to balance the subtle-body system and its components—srotas, doshas, vayus, nadis, and chakras. The strokes are done with gentle pressure, away from the heart to enhance arterial blood flow into the muscles and organ systems. The physical sheath (annamaya kosha) benefits from improved srota circulation, resulting in greater physical function. While all srotas are benefited by abhyanga, the srotas that are most cleared by the LifeSpa abhyanga are:

- Pranavaha srotas—moving prana away from the heart into the circulatory system.
- Annavaha srotas—because all abhyanga strokes are basically away from the heart, the effect is moving nourishment from the digestive system to the dhatus (tissues). The following list describes which srotas are most supported by abhyanga:
  - Raktavaha srotas—enhance blood carrying channels.
  - Mamsavaha srotas—move channels that support the muscular system.
  - Medavaha srotas—move channels that nourish fat cells.
  - Majjavaha srotas—move channels that nourish the nervous system.

- Shukravaha srotas—support the reproductive system.
- Svedavaha srotas—because abhyanga uses heated and herbalized oils, it facilitates detoxification through the sweat glands.
- Purishavaha and mutravaha srotas—because of the downward direction of most strokes, apana vata is stimulated, activating eliminative channels.
- Manovaha srotas—because of the unique nature of each stroke described in Chapter 5, the vayus are properly stimulated, resulting in nadi activation, which supports the manomaya kosha (mental sheath). This effect is described in detail in Chapter 3.

In the energy sheath (pranamaya kosha), abyhanga specifically activates the vayus and nadis. The circular strokes on the joints; long, full-handed strokes over the long bones; and spiraling strokes over the chest and abdomen are designed to move vayus, activate nadis, and illuminate chakras. While all ten vayus are benefited by abhyanga, the five main vayus are directly affected. In the same way, most nadis are gently activated with abhyanga through the movement of the vayus. Refer to Chapter 5 for details on the effects of individual strokes.

According to Vagbhata in the major Ayurvedic text *Astanga Hridaya,* effects of abhyanga are:

- Prevents and corrects the aging process
- Overcomes fatigue
- Prevents and corrects affliction of the nervous system
- Promotes better eyesight
- Nourishes the body
- Promotes longevity
- Improves sleep
- Promotes sturdiness of the body

In the *Caraka Samhita,* the other major Ayurvedic text, Ayurvedic massage as a form of snehana is said to be like a pot smeared with oil—impurities of Vata, Pitta and Kapha cannot stick to it. In the same way, if the body is properly oiled with daily Ayurvedic massage, impurities cannot penetrate and disease cannot ensue.

Abhyanga:
Best time of day: Before bathing
Frequency: Daily
Body type: All body types

One-Therapist Abyhanga
2 Positions
30–35 Minutes

Purpose
Abhyanga is an herbal-oil massage that stimulates both arterial and lymphatic circulation, enlivening and revitalizing the body.

Massage Technique
Moderate pressure according to constitution is used. Lighten pressure over face, neck, sternum, gastrointestinal region, and kidneys. Apply sufficient oil to lubricate skin, and massage slowly and rhythmically. Strokes are up and down on extremities.

Head Preparation: Position 1

Guest Position: Lying supine.
Therapist Position: Head of table.

- Oil face and scalp.
- Karna Purana (optional: see Chapter 5, p. 56): Oil both ears. Turn head to one side. Fill ear canal and massage lymph 1 minute. Place cotton ball into ear to keep oil in. Repeat on other side.

Head Preparation: Position 2

Guest Position: Ask guest to sit up. Legs can be crossed, straight out, or off table.

Therapist Position: Right side of table. Therapist can use step stool if necessary to reach head.

Head

- Pour one tablespoon oil over simanta marma.

- Marma therapy for 15 seconds with extremely light touch.
- Repeat on adhipati marma.

- Four light strokes over both marmas.

- Hand strokes on side/back of scalp for 45 seconds.

- Turn head straight and do strokes on top of head 45 seconds.

- With final stroke, smooth and tie up hair if needed.

Back

Oil spine.

- Three sets of five Seat of Vata circles and up spine with one hand.

- Finish with gentle occipital lift.

- While holding occiput, help guest lie down.

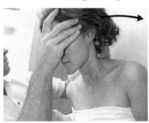

Two-Position Abhyanga—One Therapist

Position 1

Guest Position: Lying supine with towel covering body. Support knees and neck as needed.

Therapist Position: Stand at head of table facing guest.

Face (See Chapter 5, pp 58–61)

- 3 face swipes
- 5 eyebrow strokes
- 5 eye circles
- 5 bridge of nose strokes
- 5 nostril circles
- 5 upper lip strokes
- 5 chin bone strokes
- 5 chin circles

- 5 cheek circles
- 5 temple circles
- 5 forehead strokes

Ears

- 10 circles up
- 10 circles down
- 10 scissors strokes

Neck

- 2 horizontal neck swipes

Face

- 3 face swipes

Body

Therapist Position: Move to right side of table. Fold towel or sheet appropriately.

- Apply warm oil to entire body
- Hello sweep

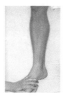 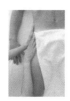 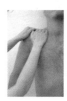

Neck

- 5 up/down cervical paraspinal finger strokes

Traps

- 5 up/down trapezius strokes

Torso (See Chapter 5, pp 80–84)

Therapist Position: Move to head of table.

- 5 down pectoral circles (women: 4 above breast and one around)
- Rest at heart—2 seconds
- 5 down pectoral circles (women: 4 above breast and one around)
- Rest at heart—2 seconds
- 5 up pectoral circles (women: 4 above breast and one around)
- Rest at heart—2 seconds
- 5 up pectoral circles (women: 4 above breast and one around)
- Rest at heart—2 seconds
- 3 down side squares—starting at midline
- 3 up side squares—ending at xiphoid process
- 5 whole torso circles
- Pause 2 seconds

Therapist Position: Move to right side of table.

- 5 heart/stomach strokes
- Rest hands on heart/stomach for 5 seconds
- Up/down/up torso butterfly stroke
- Follow through to hand, then back up to shoulder

Arm (Three planes are addressed individually. Strokes are up and down—one hand may be used to stabilize guest by holding wrist.)

Outside Plane

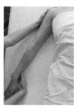

Therapist Position: Right side of table, facing guest's head.

- 3 shoulder circles up and out
- 5 upper arm strokes
- 3 elbow circles
- 5 forearm strokes
- 3 wrist circles
- Follow off hand and sweep up arm

Top Plane

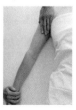

Therapist Position: Right side of table, facing guest.

- 3 shoulder circles up and in
- 5 upper arm strokes
- 3 elbow circles
- 5 forearm strokes
- 3 wrist circles
- Follow off hand and sweep up arm

Inside Plane (rotate arm laterally, palm up)

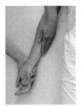

Therapist Position: Right side of table, facing guest's feet.

- 5 upper arm strokes
- 3 elbow circles
- 5 forearm strokes
- 3 wrist circles
- Follow off hand

Hand (bend arm at elbow, See Chapter 5, pp 78–79)

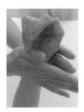

- 30 bicycle wrist circles
- Follow down to fingers
- 5 pumping heart strokes
- 30 bicycle hand circles
- Follow down to fingers
- Milk fingers
- 10 alternating squeezes
- Follow off hand
- Lay arm on table
- One-handed sweep up arm to shoulder and back down to hand
- Goodbye arm sweep
- Sweep back up from foot to hip

Leg (Three planes are addressed individually. Strokes are up and down—both hands may be needed for larger guests. See Chapter 5, pp 84–89)

Outside Plane

Therapist Position: Right side of table facing guest's head.

- 3 hip circles up and out
- 5 upper leg strokes
- 3 knee circles
- 5 calf strokes
- 3 ankle circles
- Follow off foot and sweep up leg

Top Plane

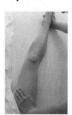

Therapist Position: Right side of table facing guest.

- 5 upper leg strokes
- 3 knee circles
- 5 calf strokes
- 3 ankle circles
- Come off foot and sweep up leg

Inside Plane

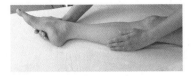

Therapist Position: Right side of table facing guest's feet.

- 5 upper leg strokes
- 3 knee circles
- 5 calf strokes
- 3 ankle circles
- Follow off foot

Foot (See Chapter 5, pp 71–77)

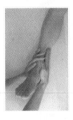

Therapist Position: Foot of table, facing guest's head.

- 30 bicycle ankle circles
- Follow through off foot
- 10 Achilles tendon strokes
- 10 thumb/heel strokes
- 10 shoeshine strokes
- 5 alternating squeezes
- Milk toes
- 30 ovals
- 10 full arch strokes
- 5 inside arch strokes
- 5 outside arch strokes
- 30 combo shoeshine/oval strokes

- Follow through off foot
- Goodbye leg
- Goodbye full-body sweep

Therapist Position: Move to left side of table and start at foot.

- Hello sweep

Repeat entire arm, hand, leg, foot, and sweep sequence on other side.

Two-Position Abhyanga—One Therapist

Position 2
Guest Position: Lying prone.
Therapist Position: Move to right side of table. Instruct guest to lie prone. Offer face cradle. Drape appropriately. If needed, place pillow under ankles.

- Apply warm oil to body
- Hello sweep, but stop at Seat of Vata instead of following all the way down legs again

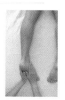 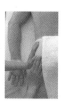

Back

- 15 Seat of Vata circles with left hand, hand up spine, occipital press

- Repeat with right hand, which follows left hand off head

Neck

- 5 up/down cervical paraspinal strokes

Traps

- 5 up/down trapezius strokes

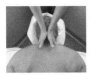

Back (See Chapter 5, pp 64–69)

Therapist Position: Stand at head of table.

- 5 down scapula circles
- Rest at heart
- 5 down scapula circles
- Rest at heart
- 5 up scapula circles
- Rest at heart
- 5 up scapula circles
- 5 up/down crescent moon strokes
- 5 up/down paraspinal strokes
- 5 up kidney circles
- 5 down kidney circles

- 5 up kidney circles
- Drop hands down to Seat of Vata
- 8 back spirals
- 2 down scapula circles
- 5 full coverage back strokes

Therapist Position: Move to right side of table.

- 2 sets of crisscross horizontal strokes
- Up/down/up butterfly strokes, follow through down arm to hand, then back to shoulder

Arm (hands cover all three planes simultaneously)
Therapist Position: Right side of table, facing guest.

- 3 outside shoulder circles (shoulder, not scapula)
- 5 upper arm strokes
- 3 elbow circles
- 5 forearm strokes
- 3 wrist circles
- Squeeze off hand
- One-handed sweep up arm, then back down to hand
- Goodbye arm sweep

Therapist Position: Move to feet.

- Two-handed sweep up leg to hip

Leg (Three planes are addressed individually. Both hands may be needed for larger guests.)

Outside Plane

Therapist Position: Right side of table facing guest's head.

- 3 hip circles up and out
- 5 upper leg strokes
- 3 knee circles
- 5 calf strokes
- 3 ankle circles
- Come off foot and sweep up leg

Top Plane

Therapist Position: Right side of table facing guest.

- 3 buttock circles up and out (hold towel/sheet)
- 5 upper leg strokes
- 3 knee circles
- 5 calf strokes
- 3 ankle circles
- Come off foot and sweep up leg

Inside Plane

Therapist Position: Right side of table facing guest's feet.

- 5 upper leg strokes
- 3 knee circles
- 5 calf strokes
- 3 ankle circles
- Come off foot

Foot (See Chapter 5, pp 71–77)

Therapist Position: Foot of table, facing guest's head.

- 30 bicycle ankle circles
- Follow through off foot
- 5 Achilles tendon strokes
- 5 combo heel squeeze/shoeshine strokes
- 3 upside-down "T" presses
- Milk toes
- 30 ovals
- 5 full arch strokes
- 5 inside arch strokes
- 5 outside arch strokes
- 10 combo shoeshine/oval strokes
- Follow through off foot
- Goodbye leg sweep
- Goodbye full-body sweep

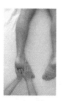
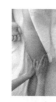
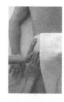
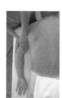
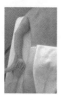

Therapist Position: Move to left side of table and start at foot.

- Hello sweep

Repeat entire arm, hand, leg, foot, and sweep sequence.

Therapist Position: When you are finished with this position cover guest back up with sheet or towel.

Wipe-Down

Done with hot, wet towels—make sure entire towel is hot, including edges.

Note: Try to cover each body part as you complete wipe-down to keep guest warm.

Towel Dip

- Fill bowl with hot water.
- Fold dry towel in half along width.
- Roll it and grab ends firmly.
- Dip middle section into hot water.
- Wring out towel and open.
- Fold dry corners into middle of towel and press.
- Open and shake towel. Test temperature on wrist. Repeat if necessary.

Note: Be sure to thoroughly cover all joints.

Therapist position: Head of table.

Face

- Towel dip.
- Lay center of unfolded towel over top half of face down to tip of nose.
- Wrap sides of towel over ears, down cheeks and jaw, and overlap ends of towel at mouth, leaving nostrils uncovered.
- Gently press towel onto forehead, cheeks and ears, and chin.
- Unfold towel from over mouth, wrap behind neck, and press gently.
- Remove towel.

Torso

Therapist Position: Side of table.

- Towel dip.
- Lay towel(s) vertically on torso.
- Press heat into chest, abdomen.
- Move towel(s) to cover as much of sides as possible and press heat in there as well.
- Remove towel(s).

Arms

- Towel dip.
- Lay one towel lengthwise from base of neck to elbow.
- Gently press.
- Move towel down to cover from elbow to fingertips.
- Lift arm slightly, wrap hands around forearm, and press down to fingers.
- Wrap towel completely around hand and press again.
- Move towel back up almost to armpit and drag and press along underside of arm down to hand.
- Remove towel while covering guest with sheet.
- Move to other arm and repeat sequence.

Legs

- Towel dip.
- Lay towel lengthwise on upper leg, starting above hip joint.
- Gently press.
- Move towel down to cover from above knee to calf and press.
- Wrap towel around foot and press.
- Lift leg slightly.
- Slide towel underneath leg; drag and press to cover as much of back surface as possible.
- Remove towel while covering guest with sheet.
- Move to other leg and repeat sequence.

Back (Ask guest to sit up.)
- Towel dip.
- Lay towel over neck and trapezius muscles and press.
- Press along spine.
- Move towel down to Seat of Vata and hold firmly to press in heat.
- Move towel to cover one side, then other, pressing heat in.
- Remove towel.

Prepare guest for next treatment.

Chapter Eight

Vishesh

Vishesh is a deep tissue form of abhyanga or Ayurvedic massage. It is of course designed as an oleation procedure, but with special impact on the musculoskeletal system. The LifeSpa vishesh strokes are slower than abhyanga strokes, using two full hands with a much deeper, constant pressure. Vishesh is designed to break up fibrous scar tissue that accumulates in the musculature as a result of excessive mental, physical, and emotional stress (see Chapter 3).

The srotas activated are all those moved by abhyanga, with a major impact on the mamsavaha, medavaha and asthivaha srotas. The vayus and nadis are not stimulated in vishesh as they are in abhyanga. Abhyanga is a subtle-body-system massage with primary impacts on the pranamaya and manomaya koshas, while vishesh works primarily on the annamaya kosha, or physical body.

This massage is better for Kapha and Pitta body types and should be used selectively for Vata body types.

One-therapist—Vishesh
3 Positions
30 minutes

Purpose
Vishesh is a deep massage that loosens impurities locked in the muscles and tissues.

Massage Technique
In general, deeper pressure is used. Lighten pressure over face, neck, sternum, gastrointestinal region, and kidneys. Little oil is applied to the body—just enough so that your hands glide smoothly, not so much that your hands feel slippery.

Head Preparation: Position 1
Guest Position: Lying supine.
Therapist Position: Head of table.

- Oil face and scalp.
- Karna Purana (optional: see Chapter 5, p. 56): Oil both ears. Turn head to one side. Fill ear canal and massage lymph 1 minute. Place cotton ball into ear to keep oil in. Repeat on other side.

Head Preparation: Position 2

Guest Position: Ask guest to sit up. Legs can be crossed, straight out, or off table.
Therapist Position: Right side of table. Therapist can use step stool if necessary to reach head.

Head (See Chapter 5, pp 55–56)
- Pour one tablespoon oil over simanta marma.
- Marma therapy for 15 seconds with extremely light touch.
- Repeat on adhipati marma.
- Four light strokes over both marmas.

- Hand strokes on side/back of scalp for 45 seconds.
- Turn head straight and do strokes on top of head 45 seconds.
- With final stroke, smooth and tie up hair if needed.

Back (See Chapter 5, pp 64–69)
- Oil spine.
- Three sets of five Seat of Vata circles and up spine with one hand.

- Finish with gentle occipital lift.

- While holding occiput, help guest lie down.

Three-Position Vishesh—One Therapist

Position 1

Guest Position: Lying supine with towel covering body. Support knees and neck as needed.
Therapist Position: Head of table facing guest.

Face (See Chapter 5, pp 58–61)

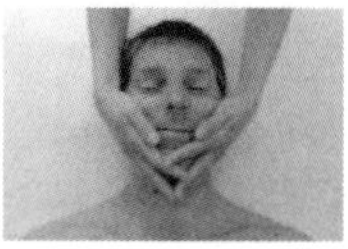

- 3 face swipes
- 5 eyebrow strokes
- 5 eye circles
- 5 bridge of nose strokes
- 5 nostril circles
- 5 upper lip strokes
- 5 chin bone strokes
- 5 chin circles
- 5 cheek circles
- 5 temple circles
- 5 forehead strokes

Ears

- 10 circles up
- 10 circles down
- 10 scissors strokes

Neck

- 2 horizontal neck swipes

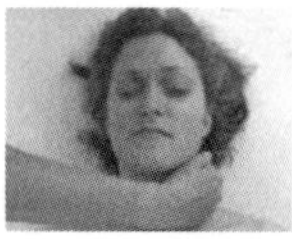

Face

- 3 face swipes

Body

Therapist Position: Move to right side of table. Fold towel or sheet appropriately.

- Apply warm oil to entire body
- Hello sweep

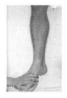

Neck

- 5 up/down cervical paraspinal strokes

Traps

- 5 up/down trapezius strokes

Torso (See Chapter 5, pp 80–84)

Therapist position: Head of table and start with right pectoral muscle.

- 5 down two-handed pectoral circles
- Rest 2 seconds at heart
- 5 down two-handed pectoral circles
- Rest 2 seconds at heart
- 5 up two-handed pectoral circles
- Rest 2 seconds at heart
- 5 up two-handed pectoral circles
- Switch to other side and repeat down and up circles

Choice of Therapist Positions:

A. Staying at head of table, do two-handed side squares with deep pressure, starting with right side, then doing left side.

or

B. Keeping hand contact with heart, move to right side of table.

- 5 two-handed down right side squares
- 5 two-handed up right side squares

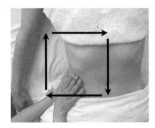

Vishesh - Side squares - from side of table

Keeping hand contact with heart, move to left side of table.

- 5 two-handed down left side squares
- 5 two-handed up left side squares

Therapist Position: Keeping hand contact with heart, move to right side of table, facing guest's head.

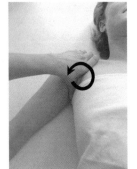

- 3 butterfly strokes
- Sweep down to right hand

Arm (hands cover all planes simultaneously)
- One-handed sweep up arm
- 3 shoulder circles (thumb in axilla)

Therapist Position: Shift body to face guest's feet.
- 5 alternating "V" pushes, upper arm
- 3 elbow circles
- 5 alternating "V" pushes, forearm

Shoulder circles

- 3 thumb circles on wrist
- Come off hand

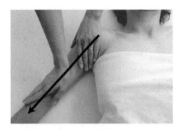

"V" pushes upper arm

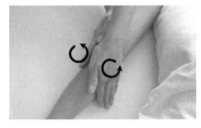

Elbow circles

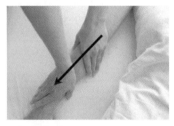

"V" pushes forearm

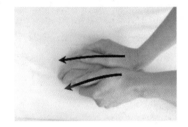

Press off of hand - supine

Hand (See Chapter 5, pp 78–79)
Therapist Position: Shift body to face guest's head.

- Milk fingers
- 5 alternating hand squeezes
- Come off hand

Arm
- One-handed sweep up arm

Therapist Position: Face guest.
- Wringing from shoulder to wrist

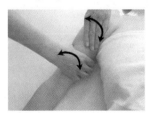

Wringing strokes on upper arm

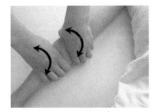

Wringing strokes on forearm

- Come off hand
- Sweep up arm
- Goodbye arm sweep

Leg (hands cover all planes simultaneously)
Therapist Position: Right side of table.
- Two-handed sweep from foot to hip

Therapist Position: Right side of table, facing guest's feet.
- 3 hip circles
- 5 alternating "V" pushes, upper leg
- 3 alternating kneecap squeezes
- 5 alternating "V" pushes, calf
- 3 ankle circles
- Come off foot

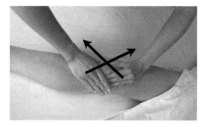

Kneecap squeezes

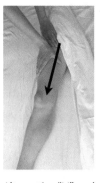

Alternating "V" pushes - legs

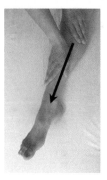

"V" pushes calf

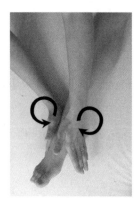

Ankle circles

Foot (See Chapter 5, pp 71–77)

Therapist Position: Foot of table, facing guest's head.

- 5 down ankle circles (hands together with pressure)
- 5 up ankle circles (hands together with pressure)
- 5 Achilles tendon strokes
- 5 thumb/heel strokes
- 5 metatarsal spreads
- Milk toes
- Come off foot

Leg (See Chapter 5, pp 84–89)

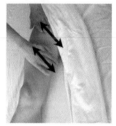

Wringing strokes

- Two-handed sweep up leg
- Wringing strokes from hip to ankle
- 5 wringing strokes on foot
- Come off foot
- Two-handed sweep up leg
- Goodbye full-body sweep

Therapist Position: Move to left side of table.
- Hello sweep

Repeat arm, hand, leg, foot, and sweep sequence.

Three-Position Vishesh—One Therapist

Position 2

Guest Position: Lying prone.
Therapist Position: Move to right side of table. Instruct guest to lie prone. Offer face cradle. Drape appropriately. If needed, place pillow under ankles.

- Apply oil to body
- Hello sweep

- Sweep down back to Seat of Vata

Back

Therapist Position: Right side of table, facing guest's head.

- 15 Seat of Vata circles with left hand, hand up spine, occipital press

- Repeat with right hand, which follows left hand off head

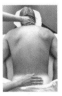

- 10 up spine strokes with thumbs

Neck/Traps
- 5 up/down cervical paraspinal strokes
- 5 up/down trapezius strokes
- 10 duck bites up neck from C7 to C1 (no down)

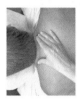

- 5 up/down strokes on neck, ending up and off neck

Back
Therapist Position: Right side of table.

- 10 down pivoting half moons on left scapula

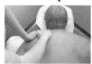

- 10 up pivoting half moons on left scapula

Therapist Position: Move to left side of table.
- Repeat up/down pivoting half moons on right scapula
- 5 two-handed up paraspinal finger strokes
- 5 two-handed down paraspinal finger strokes
- 2 sets alternating pulls across back from hip to shoulders to hip

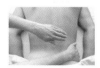

Therapist Position: Move to right side of table using hand on heart transition.
- 2 sets alternating pulls across back from hip to shoulders to hip

Therapist Position: Go to head of table.

- 3 side pulls (both sides at once)

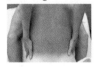

- Follow down left arm to hand

Arm (hands cover all planes simultaneously)
Therapist Position: Facing guest, except on sweeps

- One-handed sweep up arm
- 3 shoulder circles (thumb in axilla)

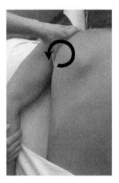

- 5 alternating "V" pushes along upper arm

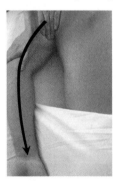

- 3 elbow circles
- 5 alternating "V" pushes along forearm
- 3 wrist circles

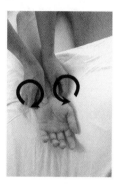

- Spread hand press

Hand

- 10 pumping heart strokes on palm

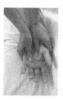

Arm

- One-handed sweep up arm
- Wringing

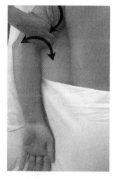

Wringing strokes on upper arm

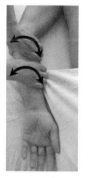

Wringing strokes on forearm

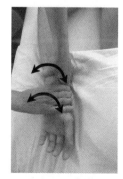

Wringing strokes on wrist

•Spread hand press

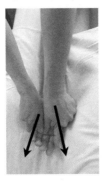

Press off hand

- Come off hand
- One-handed sweep up arm
- Goodbye arm sweep

Therapist Position: Right side of table, facing guest's feet, except on sweeps.
- Two-handed sweep from foot to hip

Buttocks
- 5 up pivoting half moons

- 5 down pivoting half moons

Leg (hands cover all planes simultaneously. See Chapter 5, pp 82–89)
- 3 hip joint circles
- 5 alternating "V" pushes along upper leg

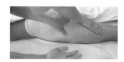

- 3 circles on knee with thenar pad
- 5 alternating "V" pushes along calf

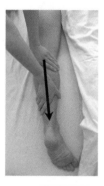

- 3 ankle circles

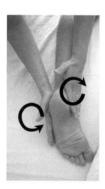

- Come off foot

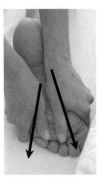

Foot (all with pressure)

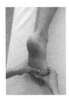

- 5 down ankle circles (hands together)
- 5 up ankle circles (hands together)
- 5 Achilles tendon strokes (hands together)
- 5 heel squeezes, cupping hands
- Upside-down "T" press
- Thumb crisscross up bottom of foot (start medially)
- Upside-down "T" press

Leg (See Chapter 5, pp 84–89)
- Two-handed sweep up leg
- Wringing strokes from hip to ankle

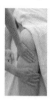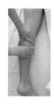

- Press off foot
- Two-handed sweep up leg
- Goodbye full-body sweep

Therapist Position: Move to left side of table.
- Hello sweep

Repeat entire arm, hand, leg, foot, and sweep sequence.

Therapist Position: When finished with this position, cover guest back up with sheet or towel. Do gentle rocking and smoothing.

Three-Position Vishesh—One Therapist

Position 3

Leg (See Chapter 5, pp 87–89)

Therapist Position: Ask guest to bend legs, still lying supine.
- Cover right foot with washcloth, sitting on right instep
- With right hand, hold knee and start at ankle with left hand
- 10 calf wrap-around strokes up

- Switch hands
- 10 calf wrap-around strokes up
- 3 calf squeezes down

- Calf press-off

Therapist Position: Move to other leg to repeat sequence.
- Cover left foot with washcloth, sitting on left instep
- With left hand, hold knee and start at ankle with right hand
- 10 calf wrap-around strokes up
- Switch hands
- 10 calf wrap-around strokes up
- 3 calf squeezes down
- Calf press-off

Wipe-Down

Done with hot, wet towels—make sure entire towel is hot, including edges.

Note: Try to cover each body part as you complete wipe-down to keep guest warm.

Towel Dip

- Fill bowl with hot water.
- Fold dry towel in half along width.
- Roll it and grab ends firmly.
- Dip middle section into hot water.
- Wring out towel and open.
- Fold dry corners into middle of towel and press.
- Open and shake towel. Test temperature on wrist. Repeat if necessary.

Note: Be sure to thoroughly cover all joints.

Therapist position: Head of table.

Face

- Towel dip.
- Lay center of unfolded towel over top half of face down to tip of nose.
- Wrap sides of towel over ears, down cheeks and jaw, and overlap ends of towel at mouth, leaving nostrils uncovered.
- Gently press towel onto forehead, cheeks and ears, and chin.
- Unfold towel from over mouth, wrap behind neck, and press gently.
- Remove towel.

Torso

Therapist position: Side of table.

- Towel dip.
- Lay towel(s) vertically on torso.
- Press heat into chest, abdomen.
- Move towel(s) to cover as much of sides as possible and press heat in there as well.
- Remove towel.

Arms

- Towel dip.
- Lay one towel lengthwise from base of neck to elbow.
- Gently press.
- Move towel down to cover from elbow to fingertips.
- Lift arm slightly, wrap hands around forearm, and press down to fingers.
- Wrap towel completely around hand and press again.
- Move towel back up almost to armpit and drag and press along underside of arm down to hand.
- Remove towel while covering guest with sheet.
- Move to other arm and repeat sequence.

Legs

- Towel dip.
- Lay towel lengthwise on upper leg, starting above hip joint.
- Gently press.
- Move towel down to cover from above knee to calf and press.
- Wrap towel around foot and press.
- Lift leg slightly.
- Slide towel underneath leg; drag and press to cover as much of back surface as possible.
- Remove towel while covering guest with sheet.
- Move to other leg and repeat sequence.

Back

Ask guest to sit up.

- Towel dip.
- Lay towel over neck and trapezius muscles and press.
- Press along spine.
- Move towel down to Seat of Vata and hold firmly to press in heat.
- Move towel to cover one side, then other, pressing heat in.
- Remove towel.

Prepare guest for next treatment.

Chapter Nine

Udvartana

Udvartana is an exfoliating lymphatic (rasa) paste massage with strokes moving only in an upward direction. The word *ud* means to go up, and together with *vartana* it means upward moving unction or oleation (snehana). The lymphatic system moves from the extremities to the heart where it drains.

The strokes are similar to abhyanga on the joints and mid-section of the body; there is an upward emphasis, with strokes usually ending on the heart.

While all the srotas are involved with this powerful therapy, rasavaha (lymph carrying), svedavaha (sweat carrying), and ambhusvaha (water regulating) srotas are most actively involved. Because a large percentage of lymph channels are layered inside and between the bellies of muscles and fat cells, the mamsavaha and medavaha channels are also very active in udvartana.

All five major vayus (located on the main lymphatic concentration points) are stimulated during udvartana. The nadis often flow toward concentrations of vayus, lymph, and nerve plexuses, so the udvartana helps activate the nadis flowing from the extremities of the body to the central command posts along the spine—the chakras. As a result, the physical, energy, and mental bodies of the subtle-body system are activated.

Benefits of Udvartana:[1]
- Removes foul smell from the body
- Cures heaviness, drowsiness, itching, skin problems, anorexia, and excessive sweating
- Balances Vata

- Balances Kapha and removes fat
- Produces stability in limbs
- Promotes skin health—good complexion
- Opens channels of circulation

Udvartana is for all body types and is usually followed by a swedana or sweat/steam therapy. Vata and Kapha types are most typically in need of this treatment.

1.   Bhagwan Dash, *Massage Therapy in Ayurveda* (New Delhi: Concept Publishing Company, 1992).

One-Therapist Udvartana
5 Positions
50 minutes

Purpose

Udvartana is an herbal paste massage specific to the lymphatic system. The massage strokes are generally done toward the heart. This massage also offers exfoliation of the skin.

Ingredients

    1½ cups Barley flour
    1½ cups Besan flour (chick-pea flour)
    2 Tbs. Bala
    2 Tbs. Mahasudarshan
    1¼ cups Sesame oil

Heat sesame oil to a very warm temperature. Pre-mix dry herbs. Mix herbs and oil together until a "peanut butter" consistency is achieved. (Note: larger guests may require increased quantities of ingredients.) Fill a large stainless steel bowl half full with hot water. Keep water on burner at low/medium setting. Place another smaller stainless steel bowl containing udvartana paste into the larger bowl of water, creating a warm water bath. Adjust temperature of burner to maintain a warm, almost hot, paste temperature.

When using udvartana paste, it should be cooled in the therapist's hands to a temperature that is experienced as hot, but not burning, by the guest. Depending on the temperature, paste can be taken from the sides of the bowl, which tend to be cooler than the middle of the bowl.

Function of Ingredients

Barley flour is granular and offers exfoliation of dead skin cells while it opens the pores.

Besan flour is an absorbent flour and acts as a "pulling" ingredient.

Bala is balancing to Vata, tones the nervous system, and is a demulcent for the skin.

Mahasudarshan is a blood purifier and tonic for the skin.

Sesame oil has anti-oxidants, vitamins and minerals, and is warming and easily absorbed.

Treatment Room Set-Up

Table: sheets, pillow, towel for head, towel to cover body, 2 or more hand towels to wipe off paste

Floor: 4 sheets to cover floor around table to protect floor/carpet if needed

Dishes: 2 stainless steel bowls (1 for water, the other for mixed paste—set paste bowl inside water bowl), 1 stainless steel cup for sesame oil, 1 mixing spoon or whisk

Massage Technique

Moderate pressure, according to constitution, is used. Lighten pressure over: face, neck, sternum, gastrointestinal region, and kidneys. Strokes are up on extremities.

Head Preparation: Position 1

Guest Position: Lying supine.
Therapist Position: Head of table.

- Oil face and scalp.
- Karna Purana (optional: see Chapter 5, p. 66): Oil both ears. Turn head to one side. Fill ear canal and massage lymph 1 minute. Place cotton ball into ear to keep oil in. Repeat on other side.

Head Preparation: Position 2

Guest Position: Ask guest to sit up. Legs can be crossed, straight out, or off table.

Therapist Position: Right side of table. Therapist can use step stool if necessary to reach head.

Head (See Chapter 5, pp 55–56)
- Pour one tablespoon oil over simanta marma.
- Marma therapy for 15 seconds with extremely light touch.
- Repeat on adhipati marma.
- Four light strokes over both marmas.

- Hand strokes on sides/back of scalp for 45 seconds.
- Turn head straight and do strokes on top of head 45 seconds.
- With final stroke, smooth and tie up hair if needed.

Back (See Chapter 5, pp 64–69)
- Oil spine with sesame oil.
- Three sets of five Seat of Vata circles, then up spine with one hand.

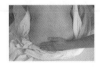
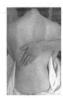

- Finish with gentle occipital lift.

- While holding occiput, help guest to lie down.

Five-Position Udvartana—One Therapist

Position 1

Guest Position: Lying supine with towel covering body.
Therapist Position: Head of table.

Face (See Chapter 5, pp 58–61)

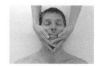

- 3 face swipes
- 5 eyebrow strokes
- 5 eye circles
- 5 bridge of nose strokes
- 5 nostril circles
- 5 upper lip strokes
- 5 chin bone strokes
- 5 chin circles
- 5 cheek circles
- 5 temple circles
- 5 forehead strokes

Ears
- 10 circles up
- 10 circles down
- 10 scissors strokes

Neck
- 2 horizontal neck swipes

Face

- 3 face swipes

Body

Therapist Position: Move to right side of table. Fold towel or sheet appropriately.

- Apply paste to entire body (make sure temperature is appropriate).
- Put paste back in hot water bath.
- Starting at foot, sweep up leg and torso to shoulder.

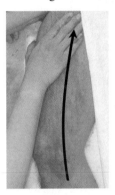

- Starting at hand, sweep up arm to shoulder.

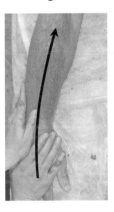

Neck
- 5 up/down cervical paraspinal strokes

Traps
- 5 up/down trapezius strokes

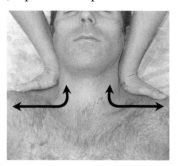

Udvartana - Up/down hand strokes along upper trapezius

Torso (See Chapter 5, pp 80–84)
- 4 sets of 5 down pectoral circles (women: 4 above breast and 1 around); after each set, rest at heart for 2 seconds
- 2 sets of 3 up side spirals
- 5 whole torso circles (starting at hips)
- Rest 2 seconds at heart

Therapist Position: Move to right side of table.
- 5 heart/stomach strokes
- Rest hands on heart/stomach for 5 seconds
- 2 up butterfly strokes
- Two-handed sweep from hand to shoulder

Arm (Three planes are addressed individually. Strokes are up—one hand may be used to stabilize guest by holding wrist.)

Outside Plane

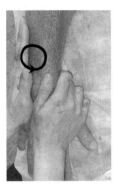

Wrist circles

Therapist Position: Right side of table, facing guest's head.
- 3 wrist circles
- 5 forearm strokes
- 3 elbow circles
- 5 upper arm strokes
- 3 outside shoulder circles up and out

Top Plane

Therapist Position: Right side of table, facing guest.
- 3 wrist circles
- 5 forearm strokes
- 3 elbow circles
- 5 upper arm strokes
- 3 inside shoulder circles up and in

Inside Plane (*rotate arm laterally, palm up*)

Therapist Position: Right side of table, facing guest's feet.

- 3 wrist circles
- 5 forearm strokes
- 3 elbow circles
- 5 upper arm strokes

Hand (bend arm at elbow. See Chapter 5, pp 78–79)
- 30 bicycle wrist circles
- Follow up to fingers
- 5 pumping heart strokes
- 30 bicycle hand circles
- Follow up to fingers
- Milk fingers
- 10 alternating hand squeezes
- Follow off hand
- Lay arm on table
- One-handed sweep from hand to shoulder
- Two-handed sweep from hand to shoulder
- Two-handed butterfly sweep up torso

Therapist Position: Move to right foot.
- Two-handed sweep from foot to hip

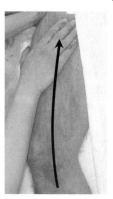

Leg (Three planes are addressed individually. Strokes are up. Both hands may be needed for larger guests. See Chapter 5, pp 84–89)

Outside Plane
Therapist Position: Right side of table, facing guest's head.

- 3 ankle circles
- 5 calf strokes

- 3 knee circles
- 5 upper leg strokes
- 3 hip circles up and out

Top Plane
Therapist Position: Right side of table, facing leg.

- 3 ankle circles
- 5 calf strokes
- 3 knee circles
- 5 upper leg strokes

Inside Plane
Therapist Position: Right side of table, facing guest's feet.

- 3 ankle circles
- 5 calf strokes
- 3 knee circles
- 5 upper leg strokes

Foot (See Chapter 5, pp 71–77)
Therapist Position: Foot of table, facing guest's head.

- 30 bicycle ankle circles
- Follow through off foot
- 5 Achilles tendon strokes
- 5 thumb/heel strokes
- 10 shoeshine strokes
- 5 alternating squeezes
- Milk toes
- 30 ovals
- 5 full arch strokes
- 5 inside arch strokes
- 5 outside arch strokes
- 30 combo shoeshine/oval strokes
- Follow through off foot
- Two-handed sweep from foot to hip

- Two-handed sweep from foot to hip again
- Two-handed butterfly sweep up torso to shoulder
- Two-handed sweep from hand to shoulder
- Follow to heart
- Rest 2 seconds

Therapist Position: Move to left side of table.
- Two-handed sweep from foot to hip
- Two-handed butterfly sweep up torso to shoulder
- Two-handed sweep from hand to shoulder

Repeat arm, hand, leg, foot, and finishing sweeps sequence.
- End at heart—rest 2 seconds

Five-Position Udvartana—One Therapist

Position 2

Guest Position: Lying on left side—bottom leg is straight and top leg is bent. Lean guest forward so back is accessible.

Therapist Position: Before guest turns, drape appropriately—turn towel from vertical to horizontal position across guest's hip. Instruct guest about position. While guest is turning, place support under head. Move to guest's back. If needed, place pillow under straight leg's foot. Move to guest's arm (facing guest's back).

- Apply paste to body
- Put paste back in hot water bath

Back (See Chapter 5, pp 64–69)
- 5 trapezius strokes
- 2 sets of 15 Seat of Vata Circles, one hand up spine

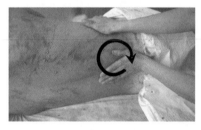

- 10 down scapula circles

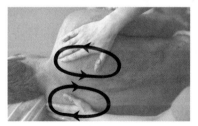

- Rest at heart
- 10 down scapula circles
- Rest at heart
- 5 up crescent moon strokes

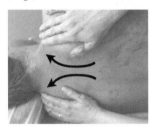

- 5 up paraspinal strokes (fingers facing head)

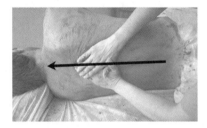

- 5 one-handed traveling up circles across kidneys

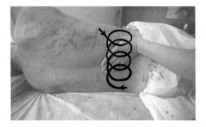

- 5 one-handed traveling down circles across kidneys
- 5 one-handed traveling up circles across kidneys
- Drop hands to Seat of Vata

- 8 back spirals
- 2 down scapula circles
- 5 up paraspinal strokes (one- or two- handed)
- 2 sets of one-handed crisscross strokes—from Seat of Vata to base of neck

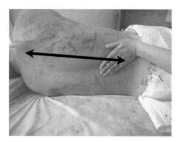

- 5 Seat of Vata circles
- Finish off neck

Therapist Position: Move to left side of table. Move guest's arm onto hip.
- One-handed sweep up arm

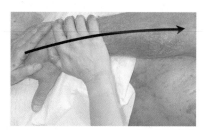

Arm (Two planes are addressed individually. Strokes are up. Both hands may be needed for larger guests. See Chapter 5, pp 86–87)

Inside Plane
- 3 wrist circles
- 5 forearm strokes
- 3 elbow circles
- 5 upper arm strokes
- 3 inside shoulder circles

Outside Plane
- 3 wrist circles
- 5 forearm strokes
- 3 elbow circles
- 5 upper arm strokes
- 3 outside shoulder circles
- Keeping arm straight with slight tension, lift off hip and forward a bit

Hand (See Chapter 5, pp 78–79)
- Milk fingers
- 5 alternating squeezes
- One-handed sweep up arm
- Bend arm at elbow
- Gently place hand (and possibly forearm) on table

Therapist Position: Move to top/bent leg.
- Two-handed sweep from foot to hip

Leg (Two planes are addressed individually. Strokes are up. Both hands may be needed for larger guests. See Chapter 5, pp 84–89)

Inside Plane
- 3 ankle circles
- 5 calf strokes
- 3 knee circles
- 5 upper leg strokes
- 3 hip circles

Outside Plane
- 3 ankle circles
- 5 calf strokes
- 3 knee circles

- 5 upper leg strokes
- 3 hip circles

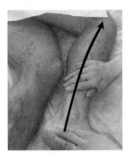

Foot (See Chapter 5, pp 71–77)
- 15 bicycle ankle circles
- Follow through off foot
- 5 Achilles tendon strokes
- 5 thumb/heel strokes
- 5 shoeshine strokes
- Follow through off foot
- Milk toes
- 15 ovals
- 5 full arch strokes
- 5 inside arch strokes
- 5 outside arch strokes
- 15 combo shoeshine/ovals
- Follow through off foot

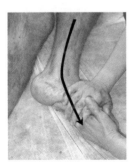

- Two-handed sweep from foot to hip
- Two-handed sweep from foot to hip, again

Therapist Position: Move to right side of table to bottom/straight leg.
- Two-handed sweep from foot to hip

Repeat leg sequence. After final foot stroke:
- Two-handed sweep from foot to bottom of towel

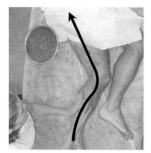

- Two-handed sweep from foot to bottom of towel, again
- From Seat of Vata, two-handed sweep up paraspinals to back of heart

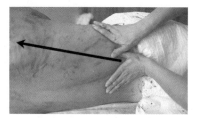

- Rest on heart 5 seconds

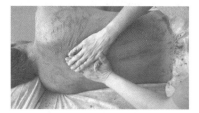

Five-Position Udvartana—One Therapist

Position 3

Guest Position: Lying prone.

Therapist Position: Drape appropriately. Instruct guest to lie prone. Offer face cradle to guest. If needed, place pillow under ankles. Move to right side of table.

- Apply paste to body. Put paste back in hot water bath.
- Start at feet, sweep up leg, up back, to shoulder

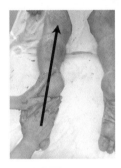 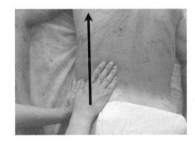

- Sweep from hand to shoulder

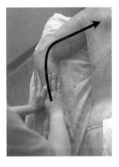

Back

Therapist Position: Right side of table.

- 15 Seat of Vata circles with left hand, up spine, occipital press
- Repeat with right hand, which follows left hand off head

Therapist Position: Head of table.

Neck (See Chapter 5, pp 62–64)
- 5 up/down cervical paraspinal strokes

Traps
- 5 up/down trapezius strokes

Back (See Chapter 5, pp 64–69)
- 2 sets of 10 down scapula circles, resting at heart after each set
- 5 up crescent moon strokes
- 5 up paraspinal strokes
- 5 up kidney circles

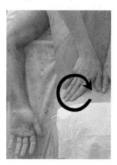

- 5 down kidney circles
- 5 up kidney circles
- Drop hands down to Seat of Vata
- 8 back spirals

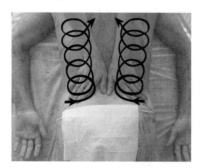

- 2 down scapula circles
- 5 paraspinal pulls

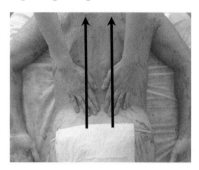

- 5 side pulls

Therapist Position: Move to right side of table.
  - 2 sets of crisscross back strokes from Seat of Vata to shoulders
  - 2 up butterfly strokes to shoulder (left side only)
  - Stabilizing arm at wrist with one hand, do one-handed sweep from hand to shoulder

Arm (hands cover all planes simultaneously See Chapter 5, pp 85–87)
Therapist Position: Right side of table, facing guest's head.

- 3 wrist circles
- 5 forearm strokes
- 3 elbow circles
- 5 upper arm strokes
- 3 shoulder (not scapula) circles
- One-handed sweep up arm to shoulder
- Two-handed sweep up arm again
- Two-handed butterfly sweep up torso

Therapist Position: Move to right foot.
  - Two-handed sweep from foot to hip

Leg (Three planes are addressed individually. Both hands may be needed for larger guests. See Chapter 5, pp 84–89)

Outside Plane
Therapist Position: Right side of table facing guest's head.

- 3 ankle circles
- 5 calf strokes
- 3 knee circles
- 5 upper leg strokes
- 3 hip circles

Top Plane
Therapist Position: Right side of table, facing guest.
- 3 ankle circles
- 5 calf circles
- 3 knee circles
- 5 upper leg strokes
- 3 hip circles (hold towel/sheet)

Inside Plane
Therapist Position: Right side of table, facing guest's feet.

- 3 ankle circles
- 5 calf strokes
- 3 knee circles
- 5 upper leg strokes

Foot (See Chapter 5, pp 71–77)
Therapist Position: Foot of table facing guest's head.

- 30 bicycle ankle circles
- Follow through off foot
- 5 Achilles tendon strokes
- 10 combo heel squeeze/shoeshine strokes
- 3 upside-down "T" presses
- Milk toes
- 30 ovals
- 5 full arch strokes
- 5 inside arch strokes

- 5 outside arch strokes
- 10 combo shoeshine/oval strokes
- Follow through off foot

- Two-handed sweep from foot to hip
- Two-handed sweep from foot to hip, continuing up torso to shoulder
- Two-handed sweep from hand to shoulder, continuing to back of heart
- Rest 5 seconds on heart

Repeat entire arm and leg sequence on other side.

Five-Position Udvartana—One Therapist

Position 4
Guest Position: Lying on right side.
Same strokes and relative positions as in Position 2

Five-Position Udvartana—One Therapist

Position 5
Guest Position: Lying supine. No more paste is applied. **Do not** massage head or feet.

Note: Paste may be drier now and a little different to massage with.

Therapist Position: Move to right side of table. Start at right foot.

- 3 foot to shoulder sweeps
- 3 hand to shoulder sweeps
- Finish and rest on heart 5 seconds

Repeat sweeps for other side and finish on heart.

Wipe Down (Done with dry towels)

Leg

- Start with foot and wipe off paste, including between toes.
- Continue up calf and upper leg.
- Bend guest's knee (tuck towel/sheet under thighs) and remove paste from underneath leg.
- Fold clean part of table sheet underneath leg before laying leg down.

Arm

- Remove paste from hand, including between fingers.
- Continue up arm.
- Bend elbow to wipe off underneath arm.
- Fold clean part of table sheet underneath arm before laying arm down.

Repeat on other side.

Torso

- Remove paste from stomach and chest using lighter pressure.

Back

- Sit guest up and remove paste from back and neck.
- Pull any paste from hair at nape of neck.

Assist guest with robe and booties, gather guest's clothing and escort them to shower. Provide washcloth, fresh towel, and new robe and booties. Start shower. Make sure there is a bathmat on the floor.

Showering Instructions

"When you take your shower do not use any soap. We have provided a washcloth that you may use to scrub off the paste. You will need to shampoo your hair at the nape of your neck. There is a clean robe and pair of booties for you to put on when you finish. You may leave the used linens in the bathroom and come back to the room for your next treatment."

PART III

Two-Person Massage Therapies

When two therapists are simultaneously massaging a client, they create a very precise bio-psychology. As the client's mind becomes confused and then gradually silenced by four synchronized massaging hands, the protective configurations of the nervous system also begin to disarm. Deeply seated toxins and stress are released, preparing the way for the subtle-body system to activate.

The dual massage transforms the body experience from a state of strain to one of calm and balance and sets up a co-existence of opposites where the mind is deeply stilled and calm yet the body is physiologically active. This paradoxical state provides the formula for healing, perfect health, and full human potential. It is the same paradox seen in nature during a hurricane, where the eye is still and the surrounding winds are active. This function is also seen in a solar system or an atom, where planets or electrons dynamically orbit around still centers. It is the human body's capacity to be tranquil at its core while simultaneously supporting limitless physical, mental, and spiritual activity.

Chapter Ten

Garshana

2 Positions
10–15 Minutes

Purpose

Garshana is a dry massage done with wool, raw silk, or terry cloth gloves. This massage is performed quickly over the skin and removes dead skin cells, stimulating the circulation and the lymphatic system. This massage can be done before any body treatment. It lasts 10 to 15 minutes and consists of two positions.

Massage Technique

This massage is performed with both hands on the body, and the hand movements are in synchrony.

Two-Position Garshana—Two Therapists

Position 1

Guest Position: Lying supine with towel covering body.
Therapist Positions: Therapist 1 on right side of table; therapist 2 on left side of table.

- Hello full-body sweep

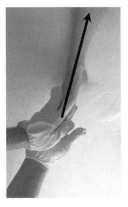

Sweep up foot

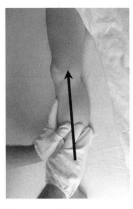

Sweep up calf

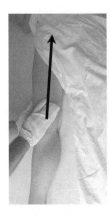

Sweep up thigh

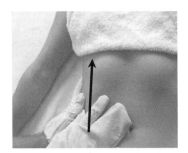

Sweep up torso

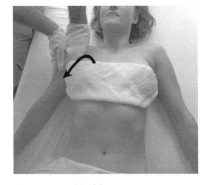

Sweep over shoulder

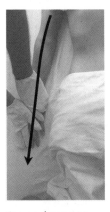

Sweep down arm

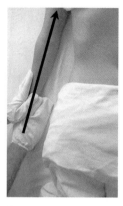

Sweep up arm

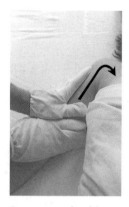

Sweep over shoulder

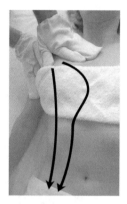

Sweep down torso

Foot

- Milk toes
- 10 toe web strokes
- 10 combo shoeshine/oval strokes
- Come off foot

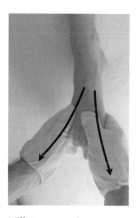

Milk toes - supine

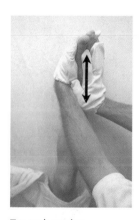

Toe web strokes

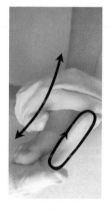

Combo shoeshine/oval
strokes

Leg (Hands cover all three planes simultaneously. Strokes are up and down, with hands moving in synchrony.)

Therapist Positions: Sides of table facing guest's head.

- 5 bicycle ankle circles
- 20 calf strokes

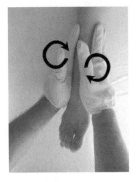 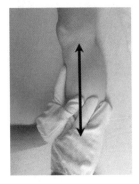

Bicycle ankle circles   Calf strokes

- 5 knee circles
- 20 upper leg strokes
- 5 one-handed hip circles

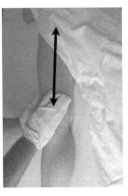 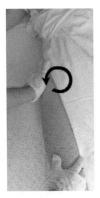

Upper leg strokes   Hip circles

Torso

- 5 up/down butterfly strokes

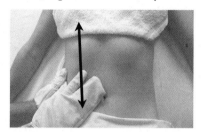

Butterfly stroke

- Follow through down to hand

Hand

- Milk fingers

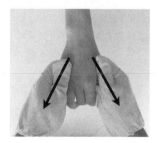

Milk fingers - beginning

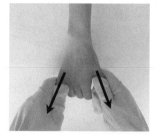

Milk fingers - pulling off fingers

- 10 finger web strokes
- 10 bicycle hand circles
- Come off hand

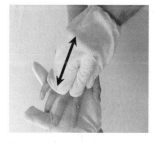

Finger web strokes

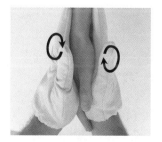

Bicycle hand circles

Arm (Hands cover all three planes simultaneously. Strokes are up and down, with hands moving in synchrony.)

Therapist Positions: Sides of table facing guest's head.
- 5 bicycle wrist circles
- 20 forearm strokes
- 5 elbow circles
- 20 upper arm strokes

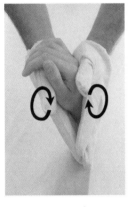 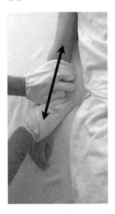 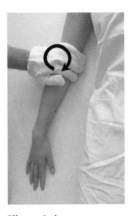 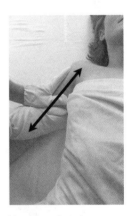

Bicycle wrist circles   Forearm strokes   Elbow circles   Upper arm strokes

- 5 two-handed shoulder circles
- Sweep down arm then back up

Therapist 1 massages face, neck, and ears.
Therapist 2 massages traps, neck, and torso.

Therapist 1
Therapist Position: Head of table.

Face
- 3 face swipes
- 5 eyebrow strokes
- 5 eye circles
- 5 bridge of nose strokes
- 5 nostril circles
- 5 upper lip strokes

- 5 chin bone strokes
- 5 chin circles
- 5 cheek circles
- 5 temple circles
- 5 forehead strokes

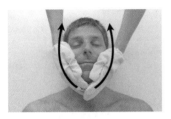

Face swipes - beginning

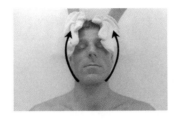

Face swipes - middle

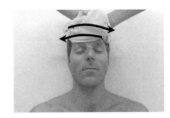

Face swipes - end

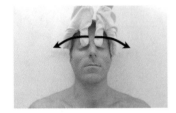

Eyebrow strokes

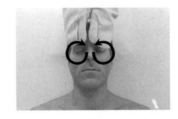

Eye circles

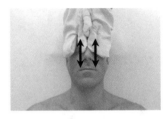

Bridge of nose strokes

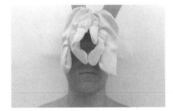

Nostril circles

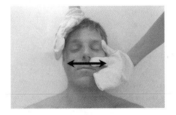

Upper lip strokes

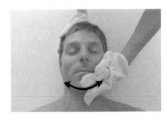

Chin bone strokes

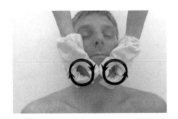

Chin circles

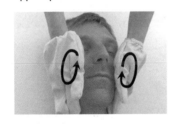

Cheek circles

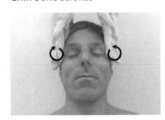

Temple circles

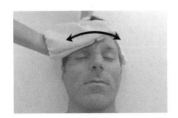

Forehead strokes

Ears

  • 10 circles up and down

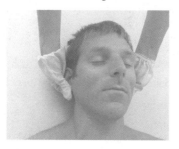

  • 10 scissors strokes

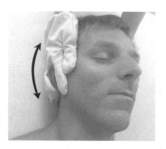

Neck

  • 10 thyroid to chin alternating neck strokes

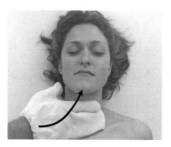

Face

- 3 face swipes
- On last face swipe both hands come off top of head

Therapist Position: Right side of table.
- Sweep down arm to fingertips
- Goodbye full-body sweep (simultaneous with Therapist 2's goodbye full-body sweep)

Therapist 2
Therapist Position: Left side of table.

Neck

- 5 up/down cervical paraspinal strokes

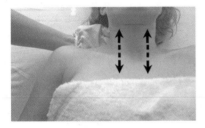

Traps

- 5 up/down trapezius strokes

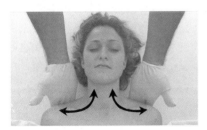

Torso

- 10 "V" strokes
- 10 upside-down "V" strokes

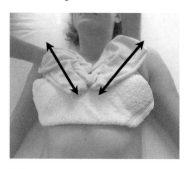

"V" strokes

Upside-down "V" strokes

- 10 up/down side strokes
- 10–20 crisscross stomach strokes (continue while waiting for Therapist 1)

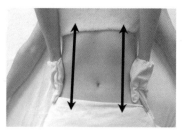
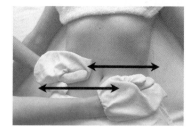

Up/down side strokes

Crisscross stomach strokes

- As Therapist 1 is completing final face sweep, come up to shoulder
- Sweep down arm to fingertips
- Goodbye full-body sweep (simultaneous with Therapist 1's goodbye full-body sweep)

Two-Position Garshana—Two Therapists

Position 2
Guest Position: Lying prone

Therapist Positions:
Therapist 1: Instruct guest to lie prone. Offer face cradle to guest. Return to right side of table.

Therapist 2: Drape appropriately. If needed, place pillow under ankles. Return to left side of table.

- Hello full-body sweep

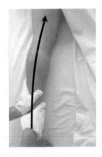
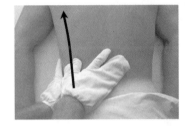
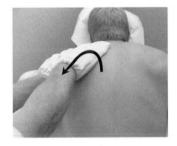

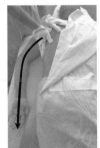
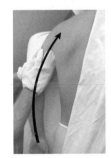
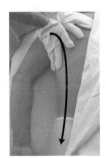
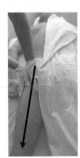

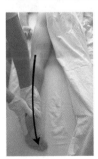

Foot
- 10 toe web strokes
- 10 combo shoeshine/oval strokes
- Come off foot

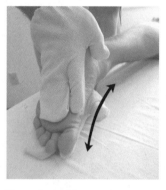

Toe web strokes

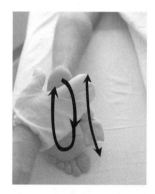

Combo shoeshine/oval (covers whole sole) strokes

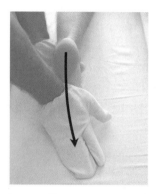

Come off foot

Leg (Hands cover all three planes simultaneously. Strokes are up and down, with hands moving in synchrony.)

Therapist Positions: Sides of table facing guest's head.
- 5 ankle circles
- 20 calf strokes

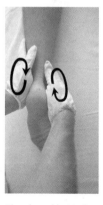

Bicycle ankle circles

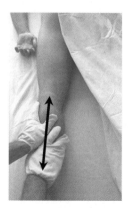

Calf strokes

- 5 knee circles
- 20 upper leg strokes
- 5 hip circles

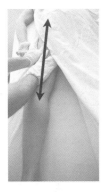   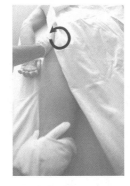

Upper leg strokes   Hip circles

Buttock

- 10 polishing circles

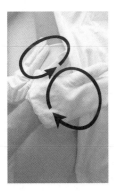

Back

- 10 up/down butterfly strokes

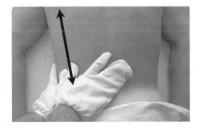

- Follow through down to hand

Arm
- 10 finger web strokes
- 5 one-handed wrist circles
- 20 forearm strokes

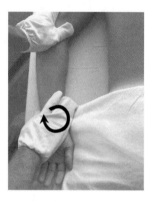

One-handed wrist circles   Forearm strokes

- 5 elbow circles
- 20 upper arm strokes
- 5 outside shoulder circles

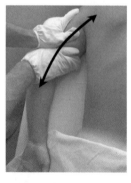 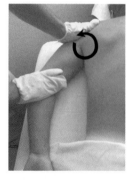

Upper arm strokes   Outside shoulder circles

- Sweep down arm
- Goodbye arm sweep
- Sweep up leg to mid-back

Back

Therapist Positions: Back is divided into two sections. Therapist 1 massages top half. Therapist 2 massages bottom half.

Therapist 1

Therapist Position: Right side of table.
- 10 "V" strokes (simultaneous with Therapist 2's upside-down "V" strokes)
- 2 sets crisscross strokes on upper back
- With Therapist 2, sweep to shoulder and down arm

Therapist 2

Therapist Position: Left side of table.
- 10 upside-down "V" strokes (simultaneous with Therapist 1's "V" strokes)
- 2 sets crisscross strokes on lower back
- With Therapist 1, sweep to shoulder and down arm

Both Therapists
- Goodbye arm sweep

Chapter Eleven

Abhyanga

4 Positions
50 minutes

Purpose
Abhyanga is an herbal-oil massage that stimulates both arterial and lymphatic circulation, enlivening and revitalizing the body.

Massage Technique
Moderate pressure according to constitution is used. Lighten pressure over face, neck, sternum, gastrointestinal region, and kidneys. Apply sufficient oil to lubricate skin, and massage slowly and rhythmically. Strokes are up and down on extremities.

Head Preparation: Position 1
Guest Position: Lying supine.
Therapist Positions: Therapist 1 at head of table—Lead Therapist; Therapist 2 at foot of table—follows lead of Therapist 1.

Therapist 1
- Oil face and scalp.
- Karna Purana (optional: see Chapter 5, p. 56): Oil both ears. Turn head to one side. Fill ear canal and massage lymph 1 minute. Place cotton ball into ear to keep oil in. Repeat on other side.

Therapist 2

- Oil feet.
- Free-form massage on feet during Therapist 1's treatment.

Head Preparation: Position 2

Guest Position: Ask the guest to sit up. Legs can be crossed, straight out, or off table.

Therapist Positions: Therapist 1 at right side of table, Therapist 2 at left side of table. Therapist can use a step stool if necessary to reach head.

Head (See Chapter 5, pp 55–56)

Therapist 1

- Pour one tablespoon oil over simanta marma.
- Marma therapy for 15 seconds with extremely light touch.
- Repeat on adhipati marma.
- Four light strokes over both marmas.

- Hand strokes on side/back of scalp for 1 minute.
- Turn head straight and do strokes on top of head 1 minute.
- With final stroke, smooth and tie up hair if needed.

Back

Therapist 2

Therapist 2 waits until Therapist 1 finishes marma points.

- When Therapist 1 begins hand strokes on head, Therapist 2 begins oiling spine

Therapists 1 & 2

- Alternate 3 sets of five Seat of Vata circles and up spine with one hand (Therapist 2 starts)

Therapist 2

- Finish with gentle occipital lift

- While holding occiput, help guest to lie down

Four-Position Abhyanga—Two Therapists

Position 1

Guest Position: Lying supine with towel covering body.
Therapist Positions: One of Therapists drapes appropriately and places pillow under knees. Therapist 1 massages head. Therapist 2 massages feet.

Head

Therapist 1

Face (See Chapter 5, pp 58–61)

- 3 face swipes
- 5 eyebrow strokes
- 5 eye circles
- 5 bridge of nose strokes
- 5 nostril circles
- 5 upper lip strokes
- 5 chin bone strokes
- 5 chin circles
- 5 cheek circles
- 5 temple circles
- 5 forehead strokes

Ears (See Chapter 5, pp 61–62)
- 10 circles up
- 10 circles down
- 10 scissors strokes

Neck
- 2 horizontal neck swipes

Face

- 3 face swipes

Feet (See Chapter 5, pp 71–77)

Therapist 2

- Oil both feet
- One foot, both hands

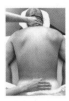

- 5 metatarsal spreads
- 5 wringing strokes
- 5 alternating squeezes
- Milk toes
- Come off foot
- Repeat on other foot
  (Watch for Therapist 1 to be finishing the face.)
- 3 finishing sweeps for feet (Strokes should be simultaneous to Therapist 1's final face sweeps. Therapists come off feet and head at same time.)

Therapist Positions: Therapist 1 moves to right side of table. Therapist 2 moves to left side of table. Strokes are done simultaneously from the two sides of the table unless otherwise indicated.

Body

- Fold towel or sheet appropriately
- Apply oil to the entire body (make sure temperature is appropriate)
- Hello sweep

Neck

- 5 up/down cervical paraspinal strokes

Traps

• 5 up/down trapezius strokes

Torso

Therapist Positions: Both therapists stand at head of table.

• 5 down pectoral circles (women: 4 above breast and one around)

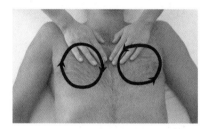

• Rest at heart—2 seconds
• 5 down pectoral circles (as in preceding)
• Rest at heart—2 seconds
• 5 up pectoral circles (as in preceding)

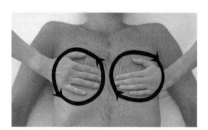

• Rest at heart—2 seconds
• 5 up pectoral circles (as in preceding)
• Rest at heart—2 seconds
• Starting at midline, move out to 3 down side squares
• 3 up side squares, ending at xiphoid process
• 5 whole torso circles (midline)
• Pause 2 seconds

Therapist Positions: Each therapist returns to own side of table.
- 5 heart/stomach strokes

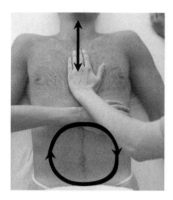

- Therapist 1—palm starts at stomach
- Therapist 2—palm starts at lower sternum
- Rest hands on heart/stomach for 5 seconds
- Up/down/up butterfly strokes
- Follow through to hand
- Sweep back up to shoulder

Arm (Three planes are addressed individually. Strokes are up and down—one hand may be used to stabilize guest by holding wrist. See Chapter 5, pp 85–87)

Outside Plane

Therapist Positions: Sides of table facing guest's head.
- 5 outside shoulder circles up and out
- 10 upper arm strokes
- 5 elbow circles
- 10 forearm strokes

- 5 wrist circles
- Come off hand and sweep up arm

Top Plane

Therapist Positions: Sides of table facing other therapist.
- 5 inside shoulder circles up and in
- 10 upper arm strokes
- 5 elbow circles
- 10 forearm strokes
- 5 wrist circles
- Come off hand and sweep up arm

Inside Plane (rotate arm laterally, palm up)

Therapist Positions: Sides of table facing guest's feet.
- 10 upper arm strokes
- 5 elbow circles
- 10 forearm strokes
- 5 wrist circles
- Come off hand

Hand (bend arm at elbow See Chapter 5, pp 78–79)

Therapist Positions: Sides of table, facing guest's head.
- 30 bicycle wrist circles
- Follow down to fingers
- 5 pumping heart strokes
- 30 bicycle hand circles
- Follow down to fingers
- Milk fingers
- 10 alternating hand squeezes
- Follow off hand
- Lay arm on table
- One-handed sweep up arm to shoulder and back again

- Goodbye arm sweep
- Sweep up to hip

Leg (Three planes are addressed individually. Strokes are up and down—both hands may be needed for larger guests. See Chapter 5, pp 84–89)

Outside Plane

Therapist Positions: Sides of table facing guest's head.
- 5 outside hip circles—up and out
- 10 upper leg strokes
- 5 knee circles
- 10 calf strokes
- 5 ankle circles
- Come off foot and sweep up leg

Top Plane

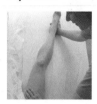

Therapist Positions: Sides of table facing other therapist.
- 10 upper leg strokes
- 5 knee circles
- 10 calf strokes
- 5 ankle circles
- Come off foot and sweep up leg

Inside Plane

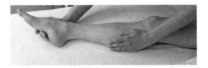

Therapist Positions: Sides of table facing guest's feet.
- 10 upper leg strokes
- 5 knee circles
- 10 calf strokes
- 5 ankle circles
- Come off foot

Foot (See Chapter 5, pp 71–77)
Therapist Positions: Foot of table facing guest's head.
- 30 bicycle ankle circles

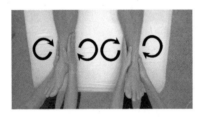

- Follow through off foot
- 10 Achilles tendon strokes
- 10 thumb/heel strokes
- 10 shoeshine strokes

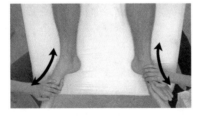

- 5 alternating squeezes
- Milk toes
- 30 ovals
- 10 full arch strokes
- 5 inside arch strokes
- 5 outside arch strokes
- 30 combo shoeshine/oval strokes
- Follow through off foot
- Goodbye leg sweep
- Goodbye full-body sweep

Four-Position Abyanga—Two Therapists

Position 2

Guest Position: Lying on left side—bottom leg is straight and top leg is bent. Lean them forward so back is accessible.

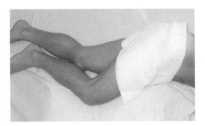

Left side position

Therapist Positions:

Therapist 1: Instruct guest about position. While guest is turning, place support under guest's head. Move to guest's back on right side of table.

Therapist 2: (before guest turns) Drape appropriately—turn towel from vertical to horizontal position across guest's hip. If needed, place pillow under straight leg's foot. Move to guest's arm at left side of table (facing guest's torso).

Both Therapists:

• Apply oil to entire body.

Therapist 1 massages back and straight leg.
Therapist 2 massages neck, shoulder, exposed arm, and bent leg.
Both therapists start and finish sequence together.

Back

Therapist 1

- 15 circles on Seat of Vata

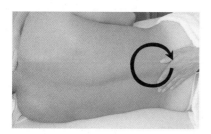

- 1 up spine sweep (signals Therapist 2 to sweep off neck)
- 1 up spine sweep (simultaneous with Therapist 2's up neck sweep)

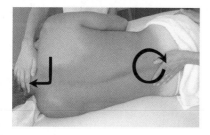

Neck/Traps

Therapist 2

While Therapist 1 is doing Seat of Vata circles:

- 5 neck/trap strokes

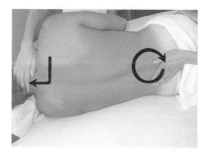
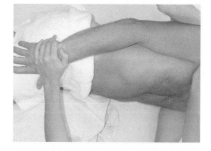

Left arm position of Therapist 2

- 1 up neck sweep (simultaneous with Therapist 1's up spine sweep)

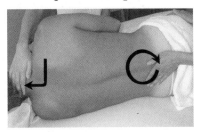

Sweep up spine - Therapists 1 & 2

Therapist Positions: Therapist 1 begins back sequence. Therapist 2 moves to arm. It is important for therapists to watch each other, as timing is tricky in this section.

Back

Therapist 1

- 5 down scapula circles

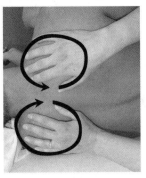

- Rest at heart
- 5 down scapula circles
- Rest at heart
- 5 up scapula circles
- Rest at heart
- 5 up scapula circles
- Rest at heart
- 5 up/down crescent moon strokes

- 5 up/down paraspinal strokes (fingers facing head)

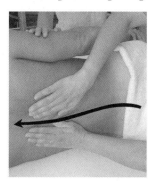

Paraspinal strokes - Therapist 1

- 5 one-handed traveling up circles across kidneys

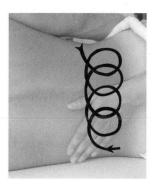

- 5 one-handed traveling down circles across kidneys
- 5 one-handed traveling up circles across kidneys
- Drop hands down to Seat of Vata
- 8 back spirals

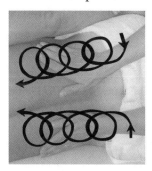

Back spirals - Therapist 1

- 2 down scapula circles
- 2 up/down back strokes along paraspinals (one- or two-handed)

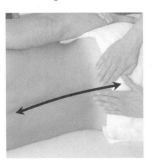

- 1 set of one-handed crisscross back strokes—from Seat of Vata to base of neck and back again
- Seat of Vata circles—watch Therapist 2 to coordinate final sweeps (With Therapist 2's final sweep up arm, finish off neck)

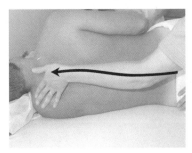

Finishing sweep off of neck - Therapist 1

Arm

Therapist 2

Therapist Position: Move guest's arm to hip.
- Sweep up from hand to shoulder
  Two planes are addressed individually.

Inside Plane

- 5 inside shoulder circles
- 10 upper arm strokes
- 5 elbow circles
- 10 forearm strokes

- 5 wrist circles
- Come off hand

Outside Plane
- 5 outside shoulder circles
- 10 upper arm strokes
- 5 elbow circles
- 10 forearm strokes
- 5 wrist circles

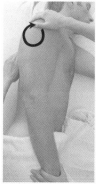 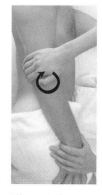 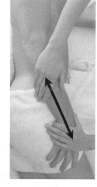 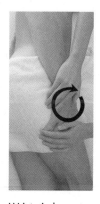 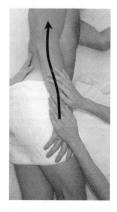

Shoulder circles   Upper arm strokes   Elbow circles   Forearm strokes   Wrist circles

- Come off hand
- Keeping arm straight with slight tension, lift off hip and forward a bit

Hand
- Milk fingers
- 5 alternating squeezes—watch Therapist 1 to coordinate final sweeps
- With Therapist 1's final neck sweep: One-handed sweep from hand to shoulder and down again

Goodbye arm sweep

- Bend arm at elbow
- Gently place hand and possibly forearm on table

Therapist Positions: Move to legs. Each therapist takes a leg.
- Sweep from hip to foot and back up to hip again

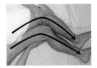

Leg
Two planes are addressed individually.

Inside Plane
- 5 inside hip circles (Therapist 1, no hip circles—wait for Therapist 2)
- 10 upper leg strokes
- 5 knee circles
- 10 calf strokes
- 5 ankle circles
- Come off foot

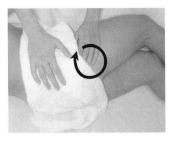

Hip circles on inside plane - Therapist 2 only

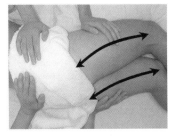

Thigh strokes on inside plane

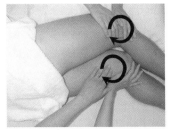

Knee circles on inside plane

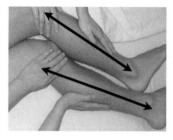

Calf strokes on inside plane

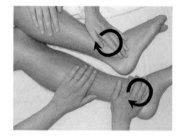

Ankle circles on inside plane

Outside Plane

- 5 outside hip circles (Therapist 1, no hip circles—wait for Therapist 2)
- 10 upper leg strokes
- 5 knee circles

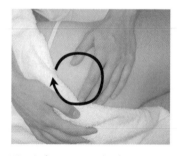

Hip circles on outside plane

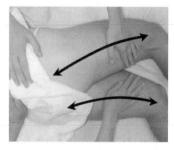

Thigh strokes on outside plane

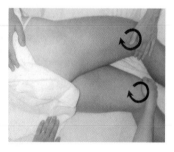

Knee circles on outside plane

- 10 calf strokes
- 5 ankle circles

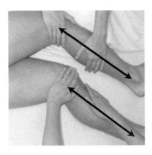 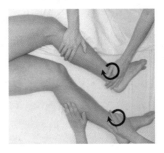

Calf strokes on outside plane   Ankle circles on outside plane

- Come off foot

Foot (See Chapter 5, pp 71–77)
- 15 bicycle ankle circles
- Follow through off foot
- 5 Achilles tendon strokes
- 5 thumb/heel strokes
- 5 shoeshine strokes
- Follow through off foot
- Milk toes
- 15 ovals
- 5 full arch strokes
- 3 inside arch strokes
- 3 outside arch strokes
- 15 combo shoeshine/oval strokes
- Follow through off foot
- Goodbye leg sweep

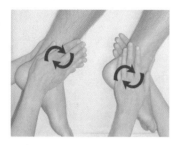

Bicycle ankle circles

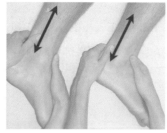

Achilles tendon strokes

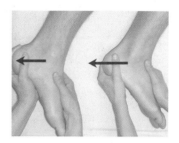

Thumb/heel strokes - side position - 2 therapists

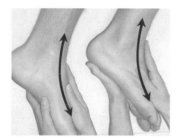

Shoeshine strokes

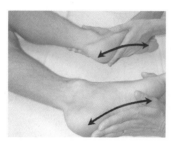

Full arch strokes

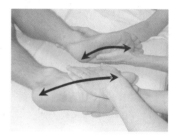

Inside arch strokes

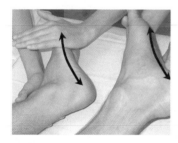

Outside arch strokes

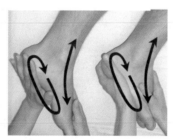

Combo shoeshine/oval strokes

Therapist 1

- Sweep up bottom leg from foot to towel
- Sweep up back starting at Seat of Vata
- With Therapist 2, rest on heart 5 seconds

Therapist 2

- Sweep up top leg from foot to hip
- Sweep up side, following rib line to mid-back
- With Therapist 1, rest on heart 5 seconds

Four-Position Abyanga—Two Therapists

Position 3

Guest Position: Lying prone.

Therapist Positions: Therapist 1: Instruct guest to lie prone. Offer face cradle to guest. Move to right side of table.

Therapist 2: Drape appropriately. If needed, place pillow under ankles. Move to left side of table.

Both Therapists:
- Apply warm oil to entire body
- Hello sweep, but stop at Seat of Vata instead of following all the way down legs again

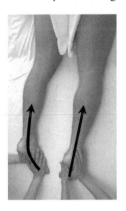 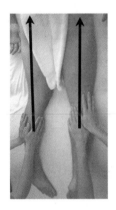 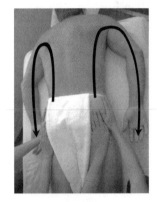

Back

Therapists 1 & 2
- Alternate 3 sets of five Seat of Vata circles, hand up spine, occipital press (Therapist 1 starts)

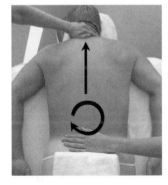

Seat of Vata circles

- As Therapist 1begins final sweep up spine, Therapist 2 sweeps off head, and Therapist 1follows

Neck and Back are done simultaneously and Traps and Sides are done simultaneously.

Neck
Therapist 1
- 5 up/down cervical paraspinal strokes

Back
Therapist 2
- 5 up paraspinal strokes

Traps
Therapist 1
- 5 up/down trapezius strokes

Sides
Therapist 2
- 5 up side strokes

Arm/Sweep
With continuity both therapists sweep down from shoulders to hands, then back up arms to scapulae. They are now ready for back sequence.

Therapist Positions: Both at head of table.

Back (See Chapter 5, pp 64–69)
- 5 down scapula circles

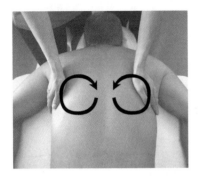

- Rest at heart
- 5 down scapula circles
- Rest at heart
- 5 up scapula circles
- Rest at heart
- 5 up scapula circles
- 5 up/down crescent moon strokes

Therapist Positions: Move to either side of guest.
- 5 up/down paraspinal strokes (fingers face other therapist)
- 5 up kidney circles
- 5 down kidney circles
- 5 up kidney circles
- Drop hands down to Seat of Vata
- 8 back spirals
- 2 down scapula circles
- 5 one-handed full coverage back strokes

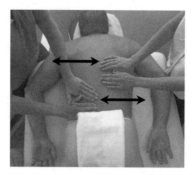

Crisscross strokes - 2 therapists

- 2 sets crisscross back strokes
- Therapist 1: from mid-back to shoulders—5 up, 5 down, 5 up, 5 down
- Therapist 2: from mid-back to Seat of Vata—5 down, 5 up, 5 down, 5 up
- Simultaneously, come off body at mid-back
- Up/down/up butterfly strokes
- Follow through down arm to hand, then back to shoulder

Arm (one plane, see Chapter 5, pp 86–87)

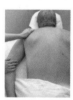

Therapist Positions: Sides of table, facing other therapist.
- 5 outside shoulder circles (shoulder not scapula)
- 10 upper arm strokes
- 5 elbow circles
- 10 forearm strokes
- 5 wrist circles
- Squeeze off hand
- Sweep up arm, then back down to hand
- Goodbye arm sweep

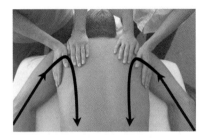

Sweep

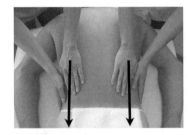

Sweep down back

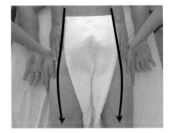

Sweep down hips and legs

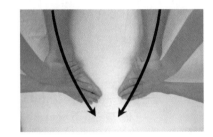

Sweep off feet

Therapist Positions: Move to feet
- Two-handed sweep up leg to hip

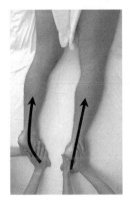

Sweep feet

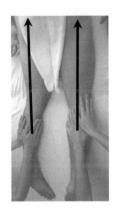

Sweep legs

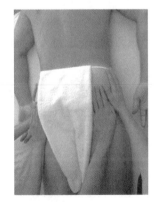

Stop at hips

Leg (Three planes are addressed individually. Both hands may be needed for larger guests. See Chapter 5, pp 84–89)

Outside Plane

Therapist Positions: Sides of table facing guest's head.
- 5 hip circles up and out
- 10 upper leg strokes
- 5 knee circles
- 10 calf strokes
- 5 ankle circles
- Come off foot and sweep up leg

Top Plane

Therapist Positions: Sides of table facing other therapist.
- 5 buttock circles up and out (hold towel/sheet)
- 10 upper leg strokes
- 5 knee circles
- 10 calf strokes
- 5 ankle circles
- Come off foot and sweep up leg

Inside Plane

Therapist Positions: Sides of table facing guest's feet.
- 10 upper leg strokes
- 5 knee circles
- 10 calf strokes
- 5 ankle circles
- Come off foot

Foot (See Chapter 5, pp 71–77)

Therapist Positions: Foot of table, facing guest's head.

- 30 bicycle ankle circles
- Follow through off foot
- 10 Achilles tendon strokes
- 10 combo heel squeeze/shoeshine strokes
- 3 upside-down "T" presses
- Milk toes
- 30 ovals
- 10 full arch strokes
- 5 inside arch strokes
- 5 outside arch strokes
- 10 combo shoeshine/oval strokes
- Follow through off foot
- Goodbye leg sweep
- Goodbye full-body sweep

Four-Position Abyhanga—Two Therapists

Position 4

Guest Position: Lying on right side (offer pillow under bent knee).

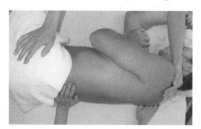

Right side position

Same as Position 2 except Therapist 1 does all of Therapist 2 strokes, and vice-versa.

Therapist Positions: When finished with this position, have guest turn onto back. Offer pillow under knees. Cover guest back up with sheet or towel.

Wipe-Down

Done with hot, wet towels—make sure entire towel is hot, including edges.

Note: Try to cover each body part as you complete wipe-down to keep guest warm.

Towel Dip
- Fill bowl with hot water.
- Fold dry towel in half along width.
- Roll it and grab ends firmly.
- Dip middle section into hot water.
- Wring out towel and open.
- Fold dry corners into middle of towel and press.
- Open and shake towel. Test temperature on wrist. Repeat if necessary.

Therapist 1 wipes down face, neck, and traps. Therapist 2 wipes down torso.

Note: Be sure to thoroughly cover all joints.

Face

Therapist 1

- Towel dip.
- Lay center of unfolded towel over top half of face down to tip of nose.
- Wrap sides of towel over ears, down cheeks and jaw, and overlap ends of towel at mouth, leaving nostrils uncovered.
- Gently press towel onto forehead, cheeks and ears, and chin.
- Unfold towel from over mouth, wrap behind neck, and press gently.
- Remove towel.

Torso

Therapist 2

- Towel dip.
- Lay towel(s) vertically on torso.
- Press heat into chest, abdomen.
- Move towel(s) to cover as much of sides as possible and press heat in there as well.
- Remove towel.

Arms

Both Therapists

Therapist Positions: Each therapist moves to one side of table.

- Towel dip.
- Lay one towel lengthwise from base of neck to elbow.
- Gently press.
- Move towel down to cover from elbow to fingertips.
- Lift arm slightly, wrap hands around forearm, and press down to fingers.
- Wrap towel completely around hand and press again.

- Move towel back up almost to armpit and drag and press along underside of arm down to hand.
- Remove towel while covering guest with sheet.

Leg
Both Therapists
- Towel dip.
- Lay towel lengthwise on upper leg, starting above hip joint.
- Gently press.
- Move towel down to cover from above knee to calf and press.
- Wrap towel around foot and press.
- Lift leg slightly (be sure both therapists are not lifting legs simultaneously, as that puts too much pressure on back).
- Slide towel underneath leg; drag and press to cover as much of back surface as possible.
- Remove towel while covering guest with sheet.

Back (Ask guest to sit up.)
One Therapist
- Towel dip.
- Lay towel over neck and trapezius muscles and press.
- Press along spine.
- Move towel down to Seat of Vata and hold firmly to press in heat.
- Move towel to cover one side, then other, pressing heat in.
- Remove towel.

Therapist 1 sets up for the following treatment.
Therapist 2 washes the dishes and cleans room.

Chapter Twelve

Vishesh

3 Positions
50 minutes

Purpose
Vishesh is a deep massage that loosens impurities locked in the muscles and tissues.

Massage Technique
In general, deeper pressure is used. Lighten pressure over: face, neck, sternum, gastrointestinal region, and kidneys. Little oil is applied to the body—just enough so that your hands glide smoothly, not so much that your hands feel slippery.

Head Preparation: Position 1
Guest Position: Lying supine.
Therapist Positions: Therapist 1 at head of table—Lead Therapist; Therapist 2 at foot of table—follows the lead of Therapist 1.

Therapist 1
- Oil face and scalp.
- Karna Purana optional (optional: see Chapter 5, p. 56): Oil both ears. Turn head to one side. Fill ear canal and massage lymph 1 minute. Place cotton ball into ear to keep oil in. Repeat on other side.

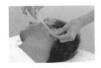

Therapist 2

- Oil feet.
- Free-form massage on feet during Therapist 1's treatment.

Head Preparation: Position 2

Guest Position: Ask guest to sit up. Legs can be crossed, straight out, or off table.

Therapist Positions: Therapist 1 at right side of table; Therapist 2 at left side of table. Therapist can use a step stool if necessary to reach head.

Head (See Chapter 5, pp 55–58)

Therapist 1

- Pour one tablespoon oil over simanta marma.
- Marma therapy for 15 seconds with extremely light touch.
- Repeat on adhipati marma.
- Four light strokes over both marmas.

- Hand strokes on side/back of scalp for 1 minute.
- Turn head straight and do strokes on top of head 1 minute.
- With final stroke, smooth and tie up hair if needed.

Back

Therapist 2

Therapist 2 waits until Therapist 1 finishes marma points.

- When Therapist 1 begins hand strokes on head, Therapist 2 begins oiling spine.

Therapists 1 and 2

- Alternate 3 sets of five Seat of Vata circles and up spine with one hand (Therapist 2 starts).

Therapist 2

- Finish with gentle occipital lift.

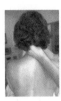

- While holding occiput, help guest to lie down.

Three-Position Vishesh—Two Therapists

Position 1

Guest Position: Lying supine with towel covering body.
Therapist Positions: Therapist 1 massages head; Therapist 2 massages feet.

Head

Therapist 1

Face (See Chapter 5, pp 58–61)

- 3 face swipes
- 5 eyebrow strokes
- 5 eye circles
- 5 bridge of nose strokes
- 5 nostril circles
- 5 upper lip strokes
- 5 chin bone strokes
- 5 chin circles
- 5 cheek circles
- 5 temple circles
- 5 forehead strokes

Ears
- 10 circles up
- 10 circles down
- 10 scissors strokes

Neck
- 2 sets of horizontal neck swipes

Face

- 3 face swipes

Feet (See Chapter 5, pp 71–77)

Therapist 2

- Oil both feet
- One foot, in both hands:
- 5 metatarsal spreads

- 5 wringing strokes
- 5 alternating squeezes
- Toes
- Repeat on other foot
  (Watch for Therapist 1 to be finishing face.)
- Both feet together:
- 3 hand strokes across top of foot

Strokes should be simultaneous to Therapist 1's final face sweeps. Therapists come off feet and head at same time.

Body

Therapist Position: Therapist 1 moves to right side of table. Therapist 2 moves to left side of table. Fold towel or sheet appropriately. Both therapists work simultaneously.

- Apply oil to entire body
- Hello sweep

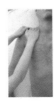

Neck
- 5 up/down cervical paraspinal strokes

Traps
- 5 up/down trapezius strokes

Torso (See Chapter 5, pp 80–84)
Therapist Positions: Both at head of table.
- 5 down two-handed pectoral circles
- Rest 2 seconds at heart
- 5 down two-handed pectoral circles
- Rest 2 seconds at heart
- 5 up two-handed pectoral circles
- Rest 2 seconds at heart
- 5 up two-handed pectoral circles
- Rest 2 seconds at heart

Therapist Positions: Stay at head of table. (Note: if guest is large, therapists may move to side of table.)
- 5 two-handed down side squares
- 5 two-handed up side squares

Therapist Positions: Move to sides of table.
- 3 butterfly strokes
- Sweep down to right hand

Arm (hands cover all planes simultaneously. See Chapter 5, pp 86–87)
Therapist Positions: Sides of table, facing head.
- One-handed sweep up arm

- 5 shoulder circles (thumb in axilla)
- 10 alternating "V" pushes, upper arm

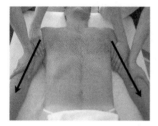

- 5 elbow circles
- 10 alternating "V" pushes, forearm
- 5 wrist circles
- Come off hand

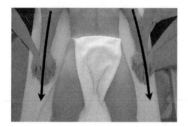

Repeat entire arm sequence.

Hand
- Milk fingers
- 5 alternating hand squeezes
- Come off hand

Arm
- Sweep up arm

Therapist positions: Face guest.
- Wringing from shoulder to wrist
- Come off hand
- Sweep up arm
- Goodbye arm sweep

Leg (hands cover all planes simultaneously. See Chapter 5, pp 84–89)
Therapist Positions: Sides of table.
- Two-handed sweep up leg

Therapist Positions: Shift body to face feet.
- 5 hip circles
- 10 alternating "V" pushes, upper leg
- 5 alternating kneecap squeezes
- 10 alternating "V" pushes, calf
- 5 alternating ankle circles
- Come off foot

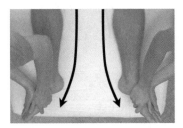

Repeat entire leg sequence.

Foot
Therapist Positions: Foot of table, facing guest's head.
- 10 down ankle circles (hands moving in synchrony, with pressure)
- 10 up ankle circles (hands moving in synchrony, with pressure)
- 10 Achilles tendon strokes
- 10 thumb/heel strokes
- 5 metatarsal spreads
- Milk toes

Leg

- Two-handed sweep up leg
- Wringing strokes from hip to ankle

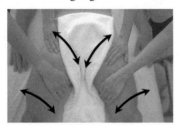

Vishesh - Wringing strokes on legs - 2 therapists

- 5 wringing strokes on foot
- Come off foot
- Sweep up leg
- Goodbye full-body sweep

Three-Position Vishnesh—Two Therapists

Position 2

Guest Position: Lying prone.

Therapist Positions: Therapist 1—instruct guest to lie prone, offer face cradle, move to right side of table. Therapist 2—drape appropriately; if needed, place pillow under ankles; move to left side of table.

Both Therapists:
- Apply oil to body

Back

Therapists 1 & 2
- Alternate 3 sets of five Seat of Vata circles, hand up spine, occipital press (Therapist 1 starts)

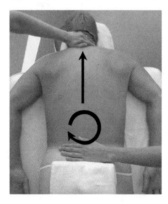

Seat of Vata circles

- As Therapist 1 begins final sweep up spine, Therapist 2 sweeps off head, and Therapist 1 follows

Therapist 1 does strokes on neck and traps while Therapist 2 does strokes up spine and sides.

Neck/Traps

Therapist 1
- 5 up/down cervical paraspinal strokes

- 5 up/down trapezius strokes
- 10 duck bites

- 5 up/down neck strokes, ending up and off neck

Back/Sides (See Chapter 5, pp 64–69)
Therapist 2
- 5 up paraspinal strokes
- 5 up side strokes
- 5 up paraspinal strokes
- 5 up side strokes

Arm
- Both therapists sweep down arm, back up to scapula

Back
- 10 down pivoting half moons
- 10 up pivoting half moons
- 5 two-handed up paraspinal finger strokes (fingers facing other Therapist)
- 5 two-handed down paraspinal finger strokes (fingers facing other Therapist)

Note: Back is now divided into 4 quadrants—upper and lower left; upper and lower right. Both therapists begin at mid-back.

Simultaneously:
Therapist 1: Upper right quadrant, standing at right side of table.
- 2 sets of alternating pulls: 5 up (mid-back to top of shoulder), 5 down (top of shoulder to mid-back)

Therapist 2: Lower left quadrant, standing at left side of table.
- 2 sets of alternating pulls: 5 down (mid-back to Seat of Vata), 5 up (Seat of Vata to mid-back)

Simultaneously:

Therapist 1: Lower right quadrant, standing at right side of table.
- 2 sets of alternating pulls: 5 down (mid-back to Seat of Vata), 5 up (Seat of Vata to mid-back)

Therapist 2: Upper left quadrant, standing at left side of table.
- 2 sets of alternating pulls: 5 up (mid-back to top of shoulder), 5 down (top of shoulder to mid-back)

Both Therapists:
- 3 butterfly strokes (up only)
- Follow down arm to hand

Arm (one plane. See Chapter 5, pp 86–87)
Therapist Positions: Facing other therapist, except on sweeps.
- One-handed sweep up arm
- 5 shoulder circles (thumb in axilla)
- 10 alternating "V" pushes along upper arm
- 5 elbow circles
- 10 alternating "V" pushes along forearm
- Spread hand press

Repeat entire arm sequence.

Hand
- 10 thumb heart circles on palm

Arm
- One-handed sweep up arm
- Wringing

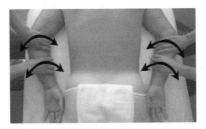

- Spread hand press
- Come off hand
- Sweep up arm
- Goodbye arm sweep

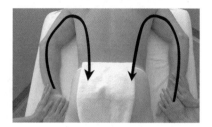 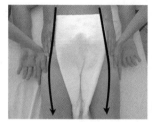 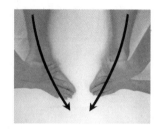

Therapist Positions: Sides of table, facing guest's feet, except on sweeps.
- Two-handed sweep up leg

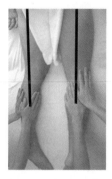

Sweep at legs - 2 therapists

Buttocks
- 5 up pivoting half moons
- 5 down pivoting half moons

Leg (hands cover all planes simultaneously. See Chapter 5, pp 84–89)
- 5 hip circles
- 10 alternating "V" pushes along upper leg

- 5 circles on knee with thenar pad
- 10 alternating "V" pushes along calf

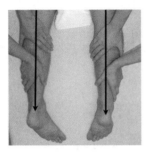

- Come off foot
- Sweep up leg
- Repeat entire leg sequence, including buttocks. Stay at foot.

Foot (See Chapter 5, pp 71–77)
- 10 ankle circles down (hands moving together, with pressure)
- 10 ankle circles up (hands moving together, with pressure)
- 10 Achilles tendon strokes
- 10 back of heel pinches
- Upside-down "T" press
- Thumb crisscross up bottom of foot (start medially)
- Upside down "T" press

Leg
- Two-handed sweep up leg
- Wringing strokes hip to ankle
- Come off foot
- Sweep up leg
- Goodbye full-body sweep

Therapist Position: When finished with this position, cover guest back up with sheet or towel. Do gentle rocking and smoothing.

Three-Position Vishesh—Two Therapists

Position 3
Leg (See Chapter 5, pp 84–89)
Guest Position: Lying supine. Ask guest to bend knees. Cover right foot with washcloth, sitting on right instep.
  • With right hand, hold knee and start at ankle with left hand.
  • 10 calf wrap-around strokes up
  • Switch hands
  • 10 calf wrap-around strokes up
  • 3 sets of calf squeezes down
  • Calf press-off

Wipe-Down
Done with hot, wet towels—make sure entire towel is hot, including edges.

Note: Try to cover each body part as you complete wipe-down to keep guest warm.

  • Towel Dip
  • Fill bowl with hot water.
  • Fold dry towel in half along width.
  • Roll it and grab ends firmly.
  • Dip middle section into hot water.
  • Wring out towel and open.
  • Fold dry corners into middle of towel and press.
  • Open and shake towel. Test temperature on wrist. Repeat if necessary.

Therapist 1 wipes down face, neck, and traps. Therapist 2 wipes down torso.

Note: Be sure to thoroughly cover all joints.

Face
Therapist 1
- Towel dip.
- Lay center of unfolded towel over top half of face down to tip of nose.
- Wrap sides of towel over ears, down cheeks and jaw, and overlap ends of towel at mouth, leaving nostrils uncovered.
- Gently press towel onto forehead, cheeks and ears, and chin.
- Unfold towel from over mouth, wrap behind neck, and press gently.
- Remove towel.

Torso
Therapist 2
- Towel dip.
- Lay towel(s) vertically on torso.
- Press heat into chest, abdomen.
- Move towel(s) to cover as much of sides as possible and press heat in there as well.
- Remove towel.

Arms
Both Therapists
Therapist Positions: Each therapist moves to one side of table.
- Towel dip.
- Lay one towel lengthwise from base of neck to elbow.
- Gently press.
- Move towel down to cover from elbow to fingertips.
- Lift arm slightly, wrap hands around forearm, and press down to fingers.
- Wrap towel completely around hand and press again.
- Move towel back up almost to armpit and drag and press along underside of arm down to hand.
- Remove towel while covering guest with sheet.

Leg
Both Therapists
- Towel dip.
- Lay towel lengthwise on upper leg, starting above hip joint.
- Gently press.
- Move towel down to cover from above knee to calf and press.
- Wrap towel around foot and press.
- Lift leg slightly (be sure both Therapists are not lifting legs simultaneously, as that puts too much pressure on back).
- Slide towel underneath leg; drag and press to cover as much of back surface as possible.
- Remove towel while covering guest with sheet.

Back (Ask guest to sit up.)
One Therapist
- Towel dip.
- Lay towel over neck and trapezius muscles and press.
- Press along spine.
- Move towel down to Seat of Vata and hold firmly to press in heat.
- Move towel to cover one side, then other, pressing heat in.
- Remove towel.

Therapist 1 sets up for the following treatment.
Therapist 2 washes the dishes and cleans room.

Chapter Thirteen

Udvartana

5 Positions
50 minutes

Purpose
Udvartana is an herbal paste massage specific to the lymphatic system. The massage strokes are generally done toward the heart. This massage also offers exfoliation of the skin.

Ingredients
    1½ cups Barley flour
    1½ cups Besan flour (chick-pea flour)
    2 Tbs. Bala
    2 Tbs. Mahasudarshan
    1¼ cups Sesame oil

Heat sesame oil to a very warm temperature. Pre-mix dry herbs. Mix herbs and oil together until a "peanut butter" consistency is achieved. (Note: larger guests may require increased quantities of ingredients.) Fill a large stainless steel bowl half full with hot water. Keep water on burner at low/medium setting. Place a smaller stainless steel bowl containing udvartana paste into the larger bowl of water, creating a warm water bath. Adjust temperature of burner to maintain a warm, almost hot, paste temperature.

When using udvartana paste, it should be cooled in the therapist's hands to a temperature that is experienced as hot, but not burning by the guest. Depending on the temperature, paste can be taken from the sides of the bowl, which tend to be cooler than the middle of the bowl.

Function of Ingredients

Barley flour is granular and offers exfoliation of dead skin cells while it opens the pores.

Besan flour is an absorbent flour and acts as a "pulling" ingredient.

Bala is balancing to Vata, tones the nervous system, and is a demulcent for the skin.

Mahasudarshan is a blood purifier and tonic for the skin.

Sesame oil has anti-oxidants, vitamins, and minerals and is warming and easily absorbed.

Treatment Room Set-Up

Table: sheets, pillow, towel for head, towel to cover body, 2 or more hand towels to wipe off paste

Floor: 4 sheets to cover floor around table to protect floor/carpet if needed

Dishes: 2 stainless steel bowls (1 for water, the other for mixed paste—set paste bowl inside water bowl), 1 stainless steel cup for sesame oil, 1 mixing spoon or whisk

Massage Technique

Moderate pressure, according to constitution, is used. Lighten pressure over face, neck, sternum, gastrointestinal region, and kidneys. Strokes are up on extremities.

Head Preparation: Position 1

Guest Position: Lying supine.

Therapist Positions: Therapist 1 at head of table—lead Therapist; Therapist 2 at foot of table—follows lead of Therapist 1.

Therapist 1

- Oil face and scalp.
- Karna Purana (optional: see Chapter 5, p. 56): Oil both ears. Turn head to one side. Fill ear canal and massage lymph 1 minute. Place cotton ball into ear to keep oil in. Repeat on other side.

Therapist 2
- Oil feet.
- Free-form massage on feet during Therapist 1's treatment.

Head Preparation: Position 2

Guest Position: Ask the guest to sit up. Legs can be crossed, straight out, or off table.

Therapist Positions: Therapist 1 at right side of table. Therapist 2 at left side of table.

Head (See Chapter 5, pp 55–56)

Therapist 1
- Pour one tablespoon over simanta marma.
- Marma therapy for 15 seconds with extremely light touch.
- Repeat on adhipati marma.
- Four light strokes over both marmas.

- Hand strokes on sides/back of scalp for 1 minute.
- Turn head straight and do strokes on top of head 1 minute.
- With final stroke, smooth and tie up hair if needed.

Back

Therapist 2

Therapist 2 waits until Therapist 1 finishes marma points.
- When Therapist 1 begins hand strokes on head, Therapist 2 begins oiling spine.

Therapists 1 & 2
- Alternate 3 sets of five Seat of Vata circles and up the spine with one hand (Therapist 2 starts).

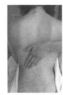

Therapist 2

- Finish with gentle occipital lift.

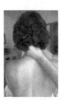

- While holding occiput, help guest to lie down.

Five-Position Udvartana—Two Therapists

Position 1

Guest Position: Lying supine with towel covering body.
Therapist Positions: Therapist 1 massages head. Therapist 2 massages feet.

Head

Therapist 1

Face (See Chapter 5, pp 58–61)

- 3 face swipes
- 5 eyebrow strokes
- 5 eye circles
- 5 bridge of nose strokes
- 5 nostril circles
- 5 upper lip strokes
- 5 chin bone strokes
- 5 chin circles
- 5 cheek circles
- 5 temple circles
- 5 forehead strokes

Ears

- 10 circles up
- 10 circles down
- 10 scissors strokes

Neck

- 2 sets of horizontal neck swipes

Face

- 3 face swipes

Feet (See Chapter 5, pp 71–77)
Therapist 2
- Oil both feet
- One foot, both hands
- 5 metatarsal spreads

- 5 wringing strokes
- 5 alternating squeezes
- Milk toes
- Repeat on other foot
- (Watch for Therapist 1 to be finishing the face.)
- 3 finishing sweeps for feet (Strokes should be simultaneous to Therapist 1's final face sweeps. Therapists come off feet and head at same time.)

Body

Therapist Positions: Therapist 1 moves to right side of table. Therapist 2 moves to left side of table. Fold towel or sheet appropriately.
- Apply paste to entire body (make sure temperature is appropriate)
- Put paste back in hot water bath

Both therapists, simultaneous strokes:
- Starting at feet, simultaneously sweep up leg and torso to shoulder
- Starting at hand, sweep up arm to shoulder

Neck
- 5 up/down cervical paraspinal strokes

Traps
- 5 up/down trapezius strokes

Torso (See Chapter 5, pp 80–84)
Therapist Positions: Both therapists at head of table.
- 4 sets of 5 down pectoral circles (women: 4 above breast and 1 around); after each set, rest at heart for 2 seconds
- 2 sets of 3 up side spirals
- 5 whole torso circles (starting at hips)
- Rest 2 seconds at heart

Therapist Positions: Each therapist returns to their side of table.
- 5 heart/stomach strokes:
- Therapist 1—palm starts at stomach
- Therapist 2—palm starts at lower sternum
- Rest hands on heart/stomach for 5 seconds
- 2 up butterfly strokes
- Two-handed sweep from hand to shoulder

Arm (Three planes are addressed individually. Strokes are up—one hand may be used to stabilize guest by holding wrist. See Chapter 5, pp 64–69)

Outside Plane
Therapist Positions: Side of table, facing guest's head.
- 6 wrist circles
- 6 forearm strokes
- 6 elbow circles
- 6 upper arm strokes
- 6 outside shoulder circles up and out

Top Plane
Therapist Positions: Side of table, facing other therapist.
- 6 wrist circles
- 6 forearm strokes
- 6 elbow circles
- 6 upper arm strokes
- 6 inside shoulder circles up and in

Inside Plane (rotate arm laterally, palm up)
Therapist Positions: Side of table, facing guest's feet.
- 6 wrist circles
- 6 forearm strokes
- 6 elbow circles
- 6 upper arm strokes

Hand (bend arm at elbow. See Chapter 5, pp 78–79)
- 30 bicycle wrist circles
- Follow up to fingers
- 5 pumping heart strokes
- 30 bicycle hand circles
- Follow up to fingers
- Milk fingers
- 10 alternating hand squeezes
- Follow off hand
- Lay arm on table
- One-handed sweep from hand to shoulder
- Two-handed sweep from hand to shoulder
- Two-handed butterfly sweep up torso

Therapist Positions: Move to feet.
- Two-handed sweep from foot to hip

Leg (Three planes are addressed individually. Strokes are up—both hands may be needed for larger guests. See Chapter 5, pp 64–69)

Outside Plane
Therapist Positions: Side of table, facing guest's head.
- 6 ankle circles
- 6 calf strokes
- 6 knee circles
- 6 upper leg strokes
- 6 hip circles up and out

Top Plane
Therapist Positions: Side of table, facing other therapist.
- 6 ankle circles
- 6 calf strokes
- 6 knee circles
- 6 upper leg strokes

Inside Plane
Therapist Positions: Side of table, facing guest's feet.
- 6 ankle circles
- 6 calf strokes
- 6 knee circles
- 6 upper leg strokes

Foot (See Chapter 5, pp 71–77)
Therapist Positions: Foot of table, facing guest's head.
- 30 bicycle ankle circles
- Follow through off foot
- 10 Achilles tendon strokes
- 10 thumb/heel strokes
- 10 shoeshine strokes
- 5 alternating squeezes
- Milk toes

- 30 ovals
- 10 full arch strokes
- 5 inside arch strokes
- 5 outside arch strokes
- 30 combo shoeshine/oval strokes
- Follow through off foot
- Two-handed sweep from foot to hip
- Two-handed sweep from foot to hip again
- Two-handed butterfly sweep up torso to shoulder
- Two-handed sweep from hand to shoulder
- Follow to heart
- Rest 2 seconds

Five-Position Udvartana—Two Therapists

Position 2

Guest Position: Lying on left side—bottom leg is straight and top leg is bent. Lean them forward so back is accessible.

Therapist Positions:
Therapist 1: Instruct guest about position. While guest is turning, place support under head. Move to guest's back at right side of table.
Therapist 2: Before guest turns, drape appropriately—turn towel from vertical to horizontal position across guest's hip. If needed, place pillow under bent leg. Move to guest's arm (facing guest's torso) at left side of table.

Both therapists:
- Apply paste to body.

Put paste back in hot water bath.
Therapist 1 massages back and straight leg.
Therapist 2 massages neck, shoulder, exposed arm, and bent leg.
Both therapists start and finish sequence together.

Back
Therapist 1
- 15 circles on Seat of Vata

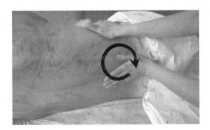

- 2 up spine sweeps (meet Therapist 2 with last neck stroke)
- Both therapists finish sweeps together with up neck stroke

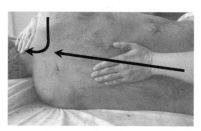 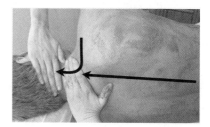

Neck/Shoulders

Therapist 2

While Therapist 1 is doing Seat of Vata circles:

- 5 trapezius strokes (meet Therapist 1 with second up spine strokes)

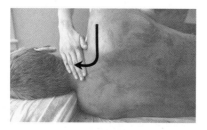

- Both therapists finish sweeps together with up neck stroke.

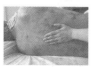

Therapist Positions: Therapist 1 begins back sequence. Therapist 2 moves to arm. It is important for therapists to watch each other, as timing is tricky in this section.

Back (See Chapter 5, pp 64–69)

Therapist 1

- 10 down scapula circles

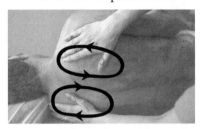

Udvartana - Down scapula circles

- Rest at heart
- 10 down scapula circles
- Rest at heart
- 5 up crescent moon strokes

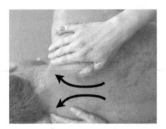

- 5 up paraspinal strokes (fingers facing head)

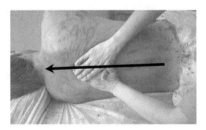

- 5 one-handed traveling up circles across kidneys

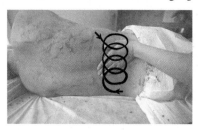

- 5 one-handed traveling down circles across kidneys
- 5 one-handed traveling up circles across kidneys
- Drop hands down to Seat of Vata
- 8 back spirals
- 2 down scapula circles
- 2 up back strokes along paraspinals (one- or two-handed)
- 1 set of one-handed crisscross back strokes—from Seat of Vata to base of neck
- Seat of Vata circles (watch Therapist 2 to coordinate final sweeps)
- With Therapist 2's final sweep up arm, finish off neck

Arm (See Chapter 5, pp 86–87)

Therapist 2

Therapist Position: Move guest's arm to hip.

- Sweep up from hand to shoulder

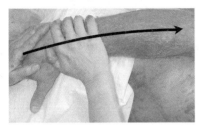

Two planes are addressed individually.

Inside Plane
- 6 wrist circles
- 6 forearm strokes
- 6 elbow circles
- 6 upper arm strokes
- 6 inside shoulder circles

Outside Plane
- 6 wrist circles
- 6 forearm strokes
- 6 elbow circles
- 6 upper arm strokes
- 6 outside shoulder circles
- Keeping arm straight with slight tension, lift off hip and forward a bit

Hand (See Chapter 5, pp 78–79)
- Milk fingers
- 5 alternating squeezes (watch Therapist 1 to coordinate final sweeps)
- With Therapist 1's final neck sweep: one-handed sweep from hand to shoulder
- Bend arm at elbow
- Gently place hand and possibly forearm on table

Therapist Positions: Move to legs. Each therapist takes a leg.

- Two-handed sweep from foot to hip

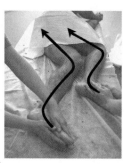

Leg (Two planes are addressed individually. See Chapter 5, pp 84–89)

Inside Plane
- 6 ankle circles
- 6 calf strokes
- 6 knee circles
- 6 upper leg strokes
- 6 hip circles

Outside Plane
- 6 ankle circles
- 6 calf strokes
- 6 knee circles
- 6 upper leg strokes
- 6 hip circles

Foot (See Chapter 5, pp 71–77)
- 15 bicycle ankle circles
- Follow through off foot
- 5 Achilles tendon strokes
- 5 thumb/heel strokes
- 5 shoeshine strokes
- Follow through off foot
- Milk toes
- 15 ovals
- 5 full arch strokes

- 5 inside arch strokes
- 5 outside arch strokes
- 15 combo shoeshine/oval strokes
- Follow through off foot

Therapist 1
- Two-handed sweep up bottom leg from foot to towel
- Two-handed sweep up bottom leg from foot to towel, again
- From Seat of Vata, two-handed sweep up paraspinals to back of heart
- With Therapist 2, rest on heart 5 seconds

Therapist 2
- Two-handed sweep up top leg from foot to hip
- Two-handed sweep up top leg from foot to hip, again
- Sweep up side, following rib line to mid-back

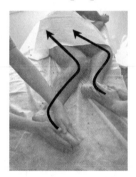 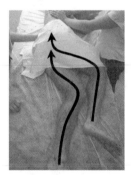

- With Therapist 1, rest on heart 5 seconds

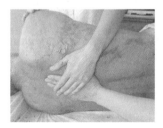

Five-Position Udvartana—Two Therapists

Position 3

Guest Position: Lying prone.
Therapist Positions:
Therapist 1: Instruct guest to lie prone. Offer face cradle to guest. Move to right side of table.
Therapist 2: Drape appropriately. If needed, place pillow under ankles. Move to left side of table.

Both therapists:

- Apply paste to body

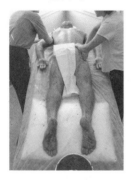

- Put paste back in hot water bath
- Starting at feet, sweep up leg, up torso to shoulder

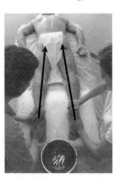

- Sweep from hand to shoulder

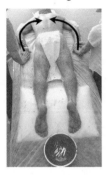

Back
Therapists 1 & 2

- Alternate 3 sets of five Seat of Vata circles, hand up spine, occipital press (Therapist 1 starts)

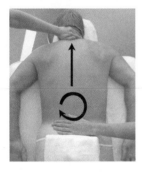

- As Therapist 1 begins final sweep up spine, Therapist 2 sweeps off head, and Therapist 1 follows

Neck and Spine are done simultaneously and Traps and Sides are done simultaneously.

Neck/Traps
Therapist 1

- 5 up/down cervical paraspinal strokes
- 5 up/down trapezius strokes

Back/Sides

Therapist 2
- 5 up paraspinal strokes
- 5 up side strokes

Arm/Sweep

With continuity both therapists sweep up arms to scapulae. They are now ready for back sequence.

Back (See Chapter 5, pp 64–69)

Therapist Positions: Both at head of table.
- 2 sets of 10 down scapula circles, resting at heart after each set
- 5 up crescent moon strokes

Therapist Positions: Move to side of table.
- 5 up paraspinal strokes
- 5 up kidney circles
- 5 down kidney circles
- 5 up kidney circles
- Drop hands down to Seat of Vata
- 8 back spirals
- 2 down scapula circles
- 5 up paraspinal strokes
- 5 up side strokes (axillary line)

- 2 crisscross back strokes
- Therapist 1: from mid-back to shoulders—up, down, up, down
- Therapist 2: from mid-back to Seat of Vata—down, up, down, up
- 2 up butterfly strokes
- 1 hand to arm stroke

Arm (Three planes are addressed simultaneously. See Chapter 5, pp 86–87)
Therapist Positions: Side of table, facing other therapist.
- 6 wrist circles
- 6 forearm strokes
- 6 elbow circles
- 6 upper arm strokes
- 6 outside shoulder circles (shoulder not scapula)

Goodbye Arm
- One-handed sweep up arm to shoulder
- Two-handed sweep back up arm
- Two-handed butterfly sweep up torso

Hello Leg
Therapist Positions: Move to feet.
- Two-handed sweep up leg to hip

Leg (Three planes are addressed individually. Both hands may be needed for larger guests. See Chapter 5, pp 84–89)

Outside Plane
Therapist Positions: Side of table facing guest's head.
- 6 ankle circles
- 6 calf strokes
- 6 knee circles
- 6 upper leg strokes
- 6 outside hip circles

Top Plane
Therapist Positions: Side of table, facing other therapist

- 6 ankle circles
- 6 calf circles
- 6 knee circles
- 6 upper leg strokes (hand position changes)
- 6 inside buttocks circles (hold towel/sheet)

Inside Plane

Therapist Positions: Side of table, facing guest's feet.

- 6 ankle circles
- 6 calf strokes
- 6 knee circles
- 6 upper leg strokes

Foot (See Chapter 5, pp 71–77)

Therapist Positions: Foot of table facing guest's head.

- 30 bicycle ankle circles
- Follow through off foot
- 10 Achilles tendon strokes
- 10 combo heel squeeze/shoeshine strokes
- 3 upside-down "T" presses
- Milk toes
- 30 ovals
- 10 full arch strokes
- 5 inside arch strokes
- 5 outside arch strokes
- 10 combo shoeshine/oval strokes
- Follow through off foot

- Two-handed sweep from foot to hip
- Two-handed sweep from foot to hip, continuing up torso to shoulder
- Two-handed sweep from hand to shoulder, continuing to back of heart
- Rest 5 seconds on heart

Five-Position Udvartana—Two Therapists

Position 4

Guest Position: Lying on right side.
  • Same as Position 2—Therapists switch massage techniques.

Five-Position Udvartana—Two Therapists

Position 5

Guest Position: Lying supine. No more paste is applied. **Do not** massage head or feet.

Note: Paste may be drier now and a little different to massage with.

Therapist Positions: Therapist 1 at right side of table. Therapist 2 at left side of table. Start at feet.
  • 3 foot to shoulder sweeps
  • 3 hand to shoulder sweeps
  • Finish and rest on heart 5 seconds

When finished with this position, cover guest back up with sheet or towel. Leave legs uncovered and start wipe-down.

Wipe-Down
(Done with **dry** towels—both therapists work simultaneously.)

Leg
  • Start with feet and wipe off paste, including between toes.

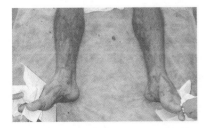

- Continue up calf and upper leg.

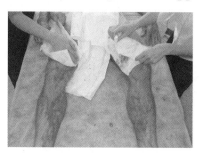

- Bend guest's knees at same time (tuck towel/sheet under thighs) and remove paste from underneath leg.

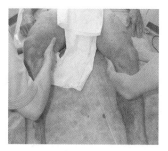

- Fold clean part of table sheet underneath leg before laying leg down.

Arm

- Remove paste from hand, including between fingers.

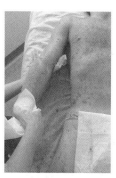

- Continue up arm.
- Bend elbow to wipe off underneath arm.

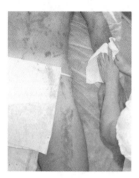

- Fold clean part of table sheet underneath arm before lying arm down.

Torso

- Remove paste from stomach and chest using lighter pressure.

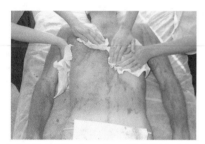

Back

- Sit guest up and remove paste from back and neck.

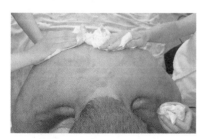

• Pull any paste from hair at nape of neck.

Therapist 1: Give showering instructions, assist guest with robe and booties, and escort them to shower. Provide washcloth, towel, and new robe and booties. Start shower. Make sure there's a bathmat on the floor.

Showering Instructions

"When you take your shower do not use any soap. We have provided a washcloth that you may use to scrub off the paste. You will need to shampoo your hair at the nape of your neck. There is a clean robe and pair of booties for you to put on when you finish. You may leave the used linens in the bathroom and come back to the room for your next treatment."

Clean-Up
Both Therapists
Therapist 1 sets up for the next treatment. While Therapist 1 assists guest with shower, Therapist 2 sweeps floor, wipes down table, washes dishes, and cleans and sets up bathroom when guest has finished showering.

PART IV

Ayurvedic Therapies That Follow Massage

There are certain Ayurvedic therapies that do not fall into the category of massage. Shirodhara, although not classically a massage, is perhaps the most important of the Ayurvedic therapies, in that it directly accesses and balances the mental body where deeply seated emotional traumas and patterns of behavior are lodged. Swedna is a fundamental therapy used in combination with Ayurvedic massage to detoxify the deepest tissues of the body. The Ayurvedic facial, while considered a beauty treatment, is also a powerful therapy used to balance the mind. Much of the body's stress is held in the head and neck, where tensions can visibly distort the contours of the face. Ayurvedic facials increase lymphatic (*rasa*) drainage in these areas, allowing the skin to function once again as an organ—restoring balance to the mind and a lively, healthy glow to the appearance.

Chapter Fourteen

Shirodhara

Shirodhara is no doubt the most popular Ayurvedic treatment in the West. The word *shiro* means head and the word *dhara* means stream. This treatment involves pouring a stream of oil over the guest's forehead. Most commonly a medicated sesame oil is used for this treatment. Traditionally, specifically prepared herbalized oils, milk, or buttermilk are used. For this book I am suggesting that pure cold-pressed (not toasted) sesame oil or herbalized sesame oil be used.

Shirodhara is one of the most powerful treatments to relieve Vata (wind) in the mind. When Vata is in excess the mind can easily become overstimulated. Preoccupied with swarming thoughts, the mind has a difficult time slowing down. This can lead to an inability to handle stress, creating nervousness, anxiety, depression, insomnia, fatigue, psychological disorders, and more. Shirodhara is the specific treatment for these disorders and any other disorder that is stress related. With eighty percent of all disease in the West now attributed to stress, shirodhara becomes one of the most important treatments in this book. Shirodhara works mainly in the manomaya kosha, or the mental sheath. It is here that the mind holds on to past impressions that create imbalanced desires (vasanas) and habitual patterns of behavior (samskaras). These impressions are held captive in the limbic system or the emotional cortex of the brain.

As oil is poured on the forehead, the nervous system is deeply stilled. The brain waves slow down and become coherent. Once the brain is quieted, the pranavaha and monovaha srotas begin to transport prana, oxygen, and other necessary nutrients to the brain. When the brain is under stress, cerebral circulation is compromised. It is in this stressed state that the ability for the brain to activate mood stabilizing receptors with the appropriate neurotransmitters is inhibited. When the brain is quieted and the srotas are activated, the cerebral circulation is greatly improved, and access to these mood stabilizing receptors is enhanced. The result: better brain function, mood stability, and improved stress handling ability. In addition, with this increase in circulatory function the mind has greater access to the limbic system where the deep seated stressors that cause emotional distortion and repetitive patterns of behavior are stored. Once the srotas bring physiological nutrition to the brain, the vayus can restore normal function. With normal vayu function the nadi system is activated, which is like turning on the master computer for the first time. From this computer control center the brain can begin to direct the spiritual process and physiological purification. Purification of the chakra system and of the physiology is effortless and efficient when directed from the master control center (the brain) rather than from organ system below.

With each successive shirodhara the mind systematically achieves an even deeper state of silence. It is like a clear alpine lake—the more still the water, the more clearly you can see the underlying imbalances (old tires, beer cans, trash…). Once the body becomes aware of the physiological problem as a problem, the healing is spontaneous. When you cut your finger you do not have to think, Scab! Scab! Scab! The healing is automatic. In the same way, when the body and mind are stilled, the mind can recognize the underlying imbalances and naturally elicit a healing response.

As the mind is deeply stilled with consecutive shirodharas, its protective layers are disarmed, giving access to stored stresses, traumas, and impressions. As the srotas are opened and the vayus are moving, the nadi system is activated. When this happens it is like a spider web weaving awareness into the different brain centers. As the brain centers open, the mind is gracefully purified, and the stress, trauma, and tension are replaced with peace, calm, and consciousness. Instead of having to relive each and every traumatic event in your life, the stress is simply softened, disarmed, and released. This often happens without specific cognitive awareness of the traumatic event but with a clear experience of a weight being lifted off the nervous system. This process is sometimes described as the soul moving through the personality. The mind, which once controlled all thoughts, actions, and desires, is gracefully replaced with the feelings and impressions felt deep in the chambers of the heart. The thinker of the thoughts is no more based on trapped emotional stress and resultant patterns of behavior but reflections of the soul expressing itself through the feelings of love and compassion from the heart. This process may take time to complete, but it is the predicted result of shirodhara.

Creating this therapeutic effect, however, is not as simple as pouring oil over your guest's head. In fact, getting the desired effect is actually a subtle yet precise process. If the oil is warmed and maintained at just the right temperature and the stream is heavy and thick from just the right height, the treatment is well begun.

The guest's comfort is crucial. The room has to be the right temperature (warm), absolutely quiet, and the neck and low back have to be supported appropriately. The oil dhara must be movable so the oil can be poured on the forehead in specific patterns determined by the guest's body type or imbalance. The type of vessel that is used can also alter the effectiveness of the treatment. Classically copper is used as it has effectiveness mostly for Vata and is also balancing for Pitta and Kapha. In our clinic we used a copper or wooden vessel for Vata, sterling silver for Pitta, and copper for Kapha. A coconut vessel is said to be one of the best and is suited for all three types. The most revered in India is a vessel made out of five metals called *pancha dhatu*. This metal is a combination of copper, nickel, brass, silver, and gold.

Shirodhara System Requirements

There are many choices to consider when purchasing a shirodhara system. I suggest that no matter what system you buy, you make sure that these four conditions are satisfied.

First, the oil stream or *dhara* should be thick and heavy, not thin and light. The dhara can be up to 1/2–inch thick. Second, the oil stream should be continuous so that if the treatment needs to last an hour, it can be provided. Be aware that some systems fill a pot with oil and when the pot runs out, the therapy is done. Be sure there is a method of refilling the shiro pot so the shirodhara can be continuous. Third, the oil needs to be warmed and needs to be maintained at just above body temperature at all times. Many systems warm the oil initially, and the oil steadily cools down as the therapy continues, sometimes leaving the oil cold by the end of the treatment. The heaviness of the oil, the warmth of the oil and the ability to effortlessly administer the shirodhara for an extended period of time are essential to disarming the protective nervous system and allowing the body to slip into a deeply relaxed healing response. The fourth component is that the stream needs to be moveable and not stationary. Oftentimes, having the oil stationary just on the third eye can be effective, but there are times when moving the oil in certain patterns is indicated. The different patterns we use are described in Chapter 5. Some spas like to set the oil over the third eye and leave the room, making treatment more cost effective. It is impossible to deliver the therapeutic effect I just described during shirodhara by leaving the client unattended.

Shirodhara—1 Therapist

30–60 minutes

Purpose
Shirodhara deeply relaxes the nervous system, lowers metabolism, integrates brain function, and creates brain wave coherence and an alpha state.

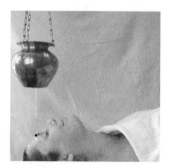

Shirodhara

Ingredients

1/2 gallon	Sesame oil (herbalized sesame oils and oil options— see Chapter 4)
5–20 drops	Essential oil (optional)

Equipment
- Table: sheets, pillow under knees, blanket, support under neck
- Oil catch (pole and cloth)
- Crockpot
- Pump with 6-inch hose attached
- Strainer
- Thermometer
- Gauze strips
- 4 cotton balls or cotton pads
- Washcloth
- Footstool

- Chair
- Clips (These are not described in the treatment—used to hold hose in place if therapist needs to pause during treatment. Also useful for maintaining hose placement as it leaves the crockpot.)

Pre-treatment set-up (this should be done before the guest arrives)

- Set up shirodhara system.

If you have a LifeSpa or other pumping shirodhara system:

- Place pump with hose attachment into crockpot.
- Add sesame oil until just covering pump.
- Place thermometer into crockpot.
- Place strainer over crockpot to filter hair.

For all systems:

- About 10 minutes before shirodhara is to start, begin heating oil. Instructions will vary with individual heating systems.
- Temperature must remain between 95 and 100 degrees. Ideal temperature is 98–99 degrees.
- Set out 2 cotton balls and gauze within reach for end of treatment.
- Select the appropriate shirodhara vessel.
- If using a pump system, attach hose to vessel with clip.
- Aim vessel to pour oil over oil catch.

Immediate set-up (this should be done just before treatment begins)

- Table: Remove face cradle, insert oil catch pole with cloth.
- Place footstool with crockpot under oil catch pole, directly under opening in cloth.
- Set chair for therapist comfort.
- Position guest face up with head tilted back slightly. Make sure guest's neck is comfortably supported.
- Explain the therapy: ("I am going to cover your eyes with cotton and gauze and then pour the oil. When I am done pouring the oil,

I will let you rest in stillness for a few moments. Then I will uncover your eyes and then you may rest for 10–15 minutes.")
- Gently place cotton over closed eyes and place gauze in 2–3 layers over eyes and around ears.
- Sit in chair and keep hose away from guest's head. Turn pump on and allow oil to begin coursing through hose. If using a vessel, allow it to fill partially up by plugging the hole with your finger.

Procedure
- Rest elbows on pad and hold vessel or hose 4–6 inches above guest's head.
- While holding vessel with both hands, slowly travel oil from top of head to third eye.
- Balance the oil on third eye.
- **Horizontal Pattern:** From third eye, gently and slowly move back and forth along the edge of the eyebrows from ear to ear. Then move the stream slightly up and repeat this motion until you are at the hairline. 3–4 horizontal lines are usually sufficient.

- **Vertical Pattern:** Gently and slowly move up and down on the forehead.

- Return to the horizontal pattern, vertical pattern, horizontal, etc.

- For Vata, stay on third eye for extended periods of time.

- For Pitta, extend horizontal pattern.
- For Kapha, extend vertical pattern and change pattern frequently.
- Final pattern should end on third eye and rest there for at least 30 seconds.
- When finished, slowly move oil from third eye to top of head, turn off the pump.
- Leave room or sit silently for 2–5 minutes.
- Remove gauze and cotton balls from eyes.
- Wipe eye region (bottom, middle, then top) with 2 clean cotton balls. Swipe across forehead from midline outward, from eyebrows to hairline.
- With 2 hands, press oil out of hair, gently squeezing hair. Continue until oil is not dripping from hair.
- With 3- to 4-inch strip of gauze, wipe forehead up to hair, following curve of head.
- Make guest comfortable: Instruct guest to move down onto table if they are uncomfortable with head tilted. Adjust pillow under knees, give blanket.
- Turn on prescribed sound therapy and leave room.
- Guest rests for 10–15 minutes.

Treatment Time: It is recommended that the Vata treatment be longer than the Pitta and the Pitta treatment be longer than the Kapha. In extreme Vata imbalances the treatment can last 60 minutes. Typically we suggest:

Vata—30–40 minutes
Pitta—25–30 minutes
Kapha—20–25 minutes

These times may be limited by guest's comfort lying on table, in which case treatment times may vary.

Put shirodhara oil into tightly sealed bottle or container and give to guest to take home to use for daily abhyanga. Be sure to tell them NOT to put this oil in their nose or mouth.

Cleaning
- Wipe excess oil off catch cloth with paper towel. Spray oil catch cloth with disinfectant.
- Use environmentally safe degreaser or cleanser of your choice.
- Oil waste: Many recycling companies will come and take your oil away at no cost.
- Remove old oil from crockpot and wipe crockpot and pump clean with paper towel. If same guest will be receiving next shirodhara treatment with this crockpot, simply refill pot with oil. If pot will be used for another guest, proceed with deep cleaning.
- Deep cleaning: Fill crockpot with soapy water and clean pot. Rinse crockpot with disinfectant. With pump in crockpot run hot water and disinfectant through pump and hose for two minutes.
- Once pump has been cleaned and new oil added, turn pump on and let oil run through into a disposable container until no longer murky (this will used approximately one cup of oil). Turn pump off again.

Caution—Fire Hazard
- Oil from shirodhara or any massage can spontaneously combust if not cared for properly.
- Oil-soiled towels and wash cloths can spontaneously combust.
- Do not wash oil-soiled towels, cloths, robes, or sheets in a standard washer and dryer as they can spontaneously combust. These linens should be sent to a professional cleaning service.
- Check with local Fire Department for recommendations on storing and cleaning oil-soiled towels, robes, sheets, and washcloths.

Chapter Fifteen

Swedana

While most Ayurvedic massage techniques fall under the classification of "nourishing" therapies, Swedana, or steam/sweat therapy, is considered "depleting." It is, however, a powerful preparatory step for the panchakarma eliminative therapies for healthy individuals. One has to use caution when administering heat therapies, particularly in Pitta aggravated conditions where swedana is mostly contraindicated.

This book is not intended for the treatment of any health conditions. Further training as a panchakarma therapist or practitioner is required for treating specific conditions. It is very important that swedana be used only for healthy individuals and after taking a thorough history. Again, any Pitta aggravation would be contraindicated for swedana.

A properly done swedana treatment can be one of the most powerful therapies in Ayurvedic massage. Unlike most steam baths, in Ayurvedic swedana the head is kept out of the steam tent; the head, heart, and lower abdomen are kept cool at all times.

If the head gets hot during a swedana, the central nervous system reacts to the heat as an emergency, at which time the entire physiology constricts. The premise of the swedana is to loosen the impurities lodged in the deep tissues of the body. The moment the body gets overheated, the treatment benefits stop. We provide a rotating ice bath on the head, heart, and lower abdomen to insure that the central nervous system stays calm and that the deep tissues remain accessible during this treatment. If the blood circulating into the brain can be maintained at a cool temperature, the nervous system will send a message to the cells of the body that it is not too hot, and it is OK to open the gates to the deep tissues to detoxify them. This process of disarming the nervous system to open up the protective tissue layers is essential in swedana. A therapist must watch this process carefully; the therapy can quickly become a failure if the client gets overheated.

As the body warms up, the entire circulatory system is stimulated, which in turn begins the flow of vayus and the activation of the nadis. Clearly the svedavaha srotas are most active in this treatment, but as the circulation accelerates, all the srotas are involved. The eliminative vayus and nadis are primarily involved in a properly done swedana.

Best time for swedana: after abhyanga, vishesh, or udvartana.

Body type: Vata and Kapha best. Pitta types—contraindicated.

SWEDANA

1 therapist
30 minutes

Purpose
Swedana is an herbalized steam bath that aids the body in releasing impurities through the sweat. The internal temperature of the body is kept cool so that the body does not experience any stress. Swedana temperature should remain at 104°–112°. Some guests can tolerate up to 120°.

Ingredients
    1 Tbs. Neem leaves
    1 Tbs. Dashamula
    Lemon oil
    Water

Function of Ingredients
Neem is primarily a blood purifier. It is also antifungal and a great skin tonic.
Dashamula is a rejuvenative aid for the nervous, reproductive and musculoskeletal systems.
Lemon essential oil is added to steam to refresh and cool the guest during the treatment
Add Vata, Pitta, or Kapha essential oils as needed.

Set-Up
- Swedana table or swedana tent set is needed.
- Fill crockpot with water and herbs.
- Prepare 1 bowl of ice and water with several washcloths. (Cold packs may also be used.)
- Lay swedana sheet on the table.
- 1 washcloth
- 1 bath towel

- 2 hand towels

Procedure

- Crockpot with herbs should be prepared at 200° during previous massage. It can be turned up to 375° just before swedana to insure proper steam. During the steam, keep crockpot at approximately 275°.
- Guest is lying face up, shoulders aligned with head of table (neck and head can be supported on face cradle). Cover their torso with large (bath-size) towel, which will be removed once swedana tent or cover is in place.

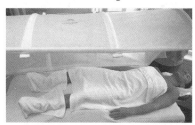

Pre-steam

- Be sure guest is covered from knees down (with either a sheet or draped hand towels).
- Wrap entire foot to protect from heat.
- Carefully place swedana tent/cover over table and guest, making sure that guest is comfortable (their head is exposed outside of tent or steam cover).

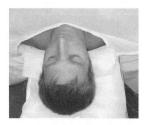

Head position

- Attach tent/cover over crockpot (crockpot should be boiling at this point with the appropriate temperature, usually 350–375°). Adjust temperature to just under 300°.
- Insert thermometer into tent/cover.
- Cover tent with solar blanket (optional).
- Constantly check temperature of tent during swedana. Do not allow tent temperature to rise above 130°.
- Instruct guest to remove towel from chest and give to therapist.
- Instruct guest to place washcloth over pubic area.
- Hand guest two ice packs—one for heart and other for pubic area, on top of washcloth.

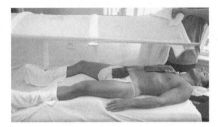

Inside tent during steam

- Cover neck opening with large bath towel that was previously covering torso.
- Place ice pack (contoured pack or crushed ice) at crown of head.
- Using icy wet towel (well wrung out), lay center of unfolded towel over top half of face down to tip of nose (top of towel will secure ice pack to crown).

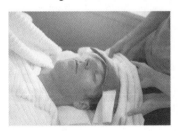

Ice on guest's head

- Wrap sides of towel over ears, down cheeks and jaw, and overlap ends of towel at mouth, leaving nostrils uncovered.

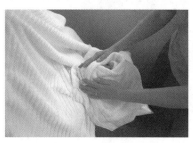

Covering guest's face

- Gently press towel onto forehead, cheeks and ears, and chin.
- Keep rotating towels (every minute or so) to insure guest stays cool. It may become more frequent as treatment progresses. REMEMBER: It is critical that guest not get overheated. Guest's comfort is of the utmost importance.
- Time can range from 15–40 minutes. Keep an eye on guest and periodically ask how they are doing. Put 3–5 drops of lemon oil into pot, through zipper as needed.
- During last 3 minutes of swedana, turn off and remove crockpot. Vent tent if possible.
- Remove thermometer.
- Ask guest to give you ice packs and washcloth and to put bath towel back onto their torso. Keep cloths on head if guest is not too cold.
- Remove wet towels and washcloths from head. Guest is now ready to rest.
- Remove tent/cover and put away.
- Cover guest with blanket if needed.
- With same towels already on legs, wipe legs dry.

Note: Guest may want to take a quick shower to rinse off sweat.

Chapter Sixteen

Ayurvedic Facial

The goal of the Ayurvedic facial is to create a deep experience of calm in both mind and body that radiates from the face. Ayurveda never intended the facial to be cosmetic, but rather transformational and permanent.

The pranavaha, manavaha, and rasavaha srotas are primarily active during the Ayurvedic facial. Strokes move lymph or rasa away from the face, initiating new blood flow and circulation to the deep layers of the skin. Prana, udana, and the first four minor vayus are activated by the facial. This treatment also stimulates nadis responsible for functions of the head and neck (see Chapter 3).

After the sequences of massage, steam, cleansers, and wrinkle therapy, the final toning mask is applied. During this period, the therapist performs an Ayurvedic hand and foot massage that promotes relaxation in every cell of the body. As an important part of the Ayurvedic experience, the facial ensures an influence on the entire central nervous system through nerve plexuses on the head, neck, and ears. The facial is, amazingly, one of the most powerful treatments in the Ayurvedic therapy menu, rivaling even shirodhara in effectiveness. It impacts the three outermost koshas — annamaya, pranamaya, and manomaya — and is good for all body types.

Ayurvedic Facial
One Therapist
50 minutes

Purpose
The goal of the Ayurvedic facial is to create a deep experience of calm in both mind and body that radiates from the face.

Equipment
- Garshana gloves
- 3 hand towels
- Crockpot filled with hot water
- Bowl filled with warm water for rinsing hands
- Eye pillow (optional)

Ingredients
Please note that this Ayurvedic facial was designed around the LifeSpa skin care line. These products are made from rejuvenative herbs with no chemicals or preservatives; the body responds to them as medicinal food. You may substitute any comparable non-preserved products of your choosing.

Cleanser-toner
Floral water mist
Herbal salve
Facial mask
Facial moisturizer
Wrinkle treatment

Abhyanga
Modified Back Sequence
Guest Position: Lying prone.
- Mix herbal salve and floral water in hand and massage into spine
- 3 full back circles

- 5 Seat of Vata circles with left hand then up spine
- 5 Seat of Vata circles with right hand then up spine and off head
- Up/down neck strokes
- Trapezius strokes
- 3 down scapula circles
- 3 up scapula circles
- 3 crescent moon strokes
- 3 up-down paraspinal strokes
- 3 up kidney circles
- 3 down kidney circles
- 5 back spirals
- 2 down scapula circles
- Reverse full back circles
- Hot towel steam and press in
- While removing hot towel cover with sheet

Guest Position: Lying supine.

Garshana
Face

- 3 face swipes
- 5 eyebrow strokes
- 5 eye circles
- 5 bridge of nose strokes
- 5 nostril circles
- 5 upper lip strokes
- 5 chin bone strokes
- 5 chin circles
- 5 cheek circles
- 5 temple circles
- 5 forehead strokes

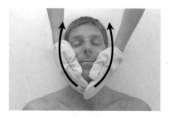

Face swipes - beginning

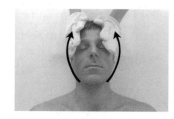

Face swipes - middle

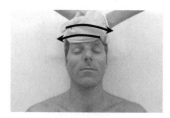

Face swipes - end

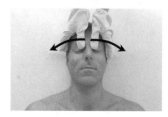

Eyebrow strokes

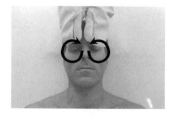

Eye circles

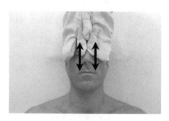

Bridge of nose strokes

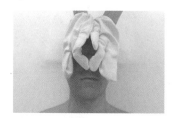

Nostril circles

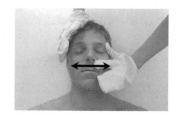

Upper lip strokes

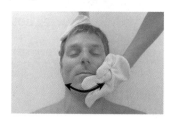

Chin bone strokes

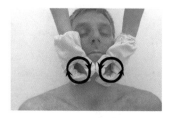

Chin circles

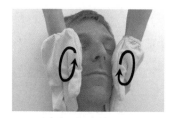

Cheek circles

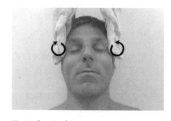

Temple circles

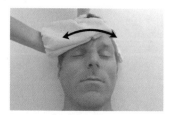

Forehead strokes

Ears

- 10 circles up

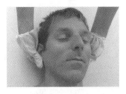

- 10 circles down
- 10 scissors strokes

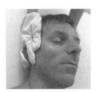

Neck

- 3 thyroid to chin alternating neck strokes

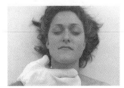

Face

- 3 face swipes

Scalp

- Remove gloves and massage scalp for 2 minutes, including occiput
- Tie hair up with clip or apply gauze around hairline, according to guest's wishes

Steam

Therapist Position: Sitting at head of table.

Towel Dip

- Fill bowl with hot water.
- Fold dry towel horizontally.
- Roll it and grab ends firmly.
- Dip middle section into hot water.
- Wring out towel and open.
- Fold the dry corners into the middle of towel and press.
- Open and shake towel. Test temperature on wrist. Repeat if necessary.

Face (can be done using three towels, with two on face at any given time and one ready to dip in hot water)

- Lay one folded towel over top half of face (going down to tip of nose and covering ears).
- Lay second folded towel from base of neck up and over mouth to just under nostrils.
- Gently press and smooth towel.

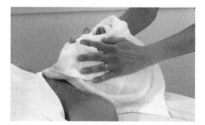

Facial steam

- As first towel starts to cool, replace with new, hot towel.

Repeat facial steam for up to 10 minutes, replacing towels as needed.

Cleanser

- Apply cleanser-toner with broad, overall strokes, then go into modified face sequence
- 3 face swipes
- 3 eyebrow strokes
- 3 eye circles
- 3 bridge of nose strokes
- 3 nostril circles
- 3 upper lip strokes
- 3 chin bone strokes
- 3 chin circles
- 3 cheek circles
- 3 temple circles
- 3 forehead strokes
- 1 final face sweep up and off face
- Wipe off with hot towels
- Apply cleanser-toner on entire face using circular finger strokes
- Rinse hands clean

Mix herbal salve and floral water mist in own hands, then begin upper torso massage.

Massage

- 3 up pectoral strokes

- 3 down pectoral strokes
- 3 side pulls

- 5 horizontal neck swipes
- 5 trapezius to occiput strokes

- Apply hot towels to upper torso
- Remove cleanser-toner with hot towels

Lymph Sequence

All strokes should be applied with thumbs, using comfortable firm pressure. Strokes move from midline to cervical lymph (just anterior to mastoid process).

Mix herbal salve and floral water mist in own hands, then apply during lymphatic drainage technique.

Lymphatic Drainage Technique

After each set of 3 strokes, use the lymphatic drainage technique: With moderate pressure, slide thumbs from cervical lymph down sides of neck to clavicle. Spread laterally across medial third of top of clavicle.

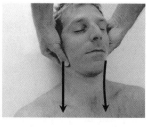 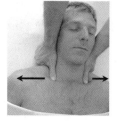

Lymph drainage - beginning   Lymph drainage - end

- 3 below chin
- 3 chin bone
- 3 below bottom lip
- 3 below maxilla
- 3 bridge of nose—above maxilla
- 3 above eyebrows
- 3 upper forehead
- 3 face swipes

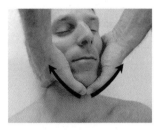

Below chin to ears

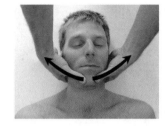

Chin bone to ears

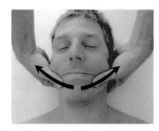

Below bottom lip to ears

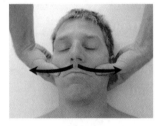

Below maxilla to ears

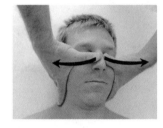

Above maxilla to ears

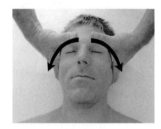

Above eyebrows to ears

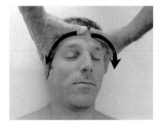

Upper forehead to ears

Repeat preceding lymph sequence.
  • 3 maxilla pulls up, hold third for 5 seconds

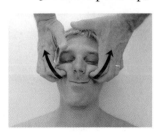

Maxilla pulls

- Sweep to cervical lymph
- Lymphatic drain
- 3 eyebrow pulls, hold third for 5 seconds

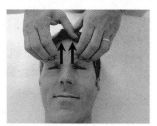

Eyebrow pulls

- Sweep across eyebrows to cervical lymph
- Lymphatic drain
- 3 face swipes

Mask

- Repeat face steam
- Apply facial mask evenly over entire face and throat
- Gently cover eyes with eye pillow (optional)
- While mask is setting (minimum 10 minutes) do hand and foot massage

Hand Massage (bend arm at elbow)

- Mix herbal salve and floral water mist in own hands, then apply to guest's hand
- 30 bicycle wrist circles

- Follow to fingers
- 5 pumping heart strokes

- 30 bicycle hand circles

- Follow to fingers
- Milk fingers
- 10 alternating squeezes

- Follow off hand
- Lay arm on table
- Repeat on other hand

Foot Massage

- Mix herbal salve and floral water mist in own hands, then apply to guest's foot
- 30 bicycle ankle circles

- Follow through off foot
- 10 Achilles tendon strokes

- 10 thumb/heel strokes

- 10 shoeshine strokes

- 5 alternating squeezes

- Milk toes
- 30 ovals

- 10 full arch strokes

- 5 inside arch strokes

- 5 outside arch strokes

- 30 combo shoeshine/oval strokes

- Follow through off foot
- Repeat on other foot

Remove Mask
- Remove mask with hot towels

Moisturizing Massage
- Mix 2–3 drops of facial moisturizer and 4 spritzes of floral water mist in own hands, then apply gently to guest's face—add more if necessary.
- Repeat lymphatic drainage technique (as described previously), but this time instead of thumb strokes, make small circles with fingertips from midline to cervical lymph as follows:

- 3 below chin
- 3 chin bone
- 3 below bottom lip
- 3 below maxilla
- 3 bridge of nose—above maxilla
- 3 above eyebrows
- 3 upper forehead

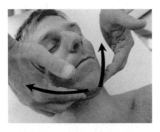

Below chin circles to ears

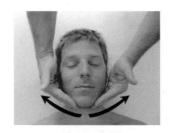

Chin bone circles to ears

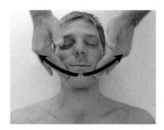

Below bottom lip circles to ears

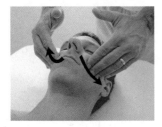

Below maxilla circles to ears

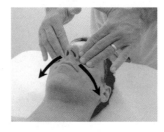

Above maxilla circles to ears

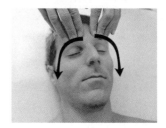

Above eyebrows circles to ears

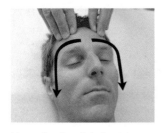

Upper forehead circles to ears

- Put 1–2 drops of wrinkle treatment on pad of own ring finger, touch to other ring finger, then apply by gently patting onto wrinkled areas.
- Gently tapote for 30 seconds, first with fingers, then with palms.
- End with final upward sweep off entire face.

Therapist leaves the room to allow approximately 5 minutes of rest.

INDEX

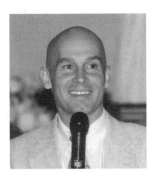

ABOUT THE AUTHOR

D
r. John Douillard began his formal Ayurvedic training in 1986 at the World Centre of Ayurveda in New Delhi, India. There he met Dr. Deepak Chopra and returned to the U.S. to co-direct his Ayurvedic Panchakarma Center for eight years. During that time Dr. Douillard became the Co-Director of the Maharishi Ayurveda Physicians Training Program where he certified Western medical doctors in Ayurvedic medicine. Dr. Douillard received extensive subsequent Ayurvedic training in India and in 1999 received his Ph.D. in Ayurvedic Medicine from the Open International University in Sri Lanka.

He is the former Director of Player Development for the New Jersey Nets Basketball Team in the NBA, where he administered chiropractic and nutritional services for two years. In 1992 Dr. Douillard published his first book, *Body, Mind, and Sport,* which has sold over 60,000 copies and is printed in six languages. In 2000 he published his second book, *The 3–Season Diet.* His first book with North Atlantic Books, *Perfect Health for Kids,* was published in 2004.

Dr. Douillard has released two audio tape series, *Invincible Athletics* and *The Ayurvedic Pulse Reading Course.* He has developed a preserva-tive-free Ayurvedic skin care line, and has recently launched an Ayurvedic herbal line for health professionals. He has been teaching Ayurveda inter-nationally for sixteen years and specializes in pulse reading, Ayurvedic fitness, and panchakarma. He recently opened the LifeSpa School of Ayurveda where he certifies massage and spa therapists in the authentic knowledge of Ayurvedic massage. Currently he practices Ayurvedic and chiropractic medicine at his LifeSpa in Boulder, Colorado, where he lives with his wife and six children.

For more information about Dr. Douillard's books, tapes, lectures and training schedule, services, and programs, please contact:

LifeSpa
PO Box 701
Niwot, CO 80544
Office: 303.516.4848
Fax: 303.530.4409
E-mail: *John@LifeSpa.com*
Website: *www.LifeSpa.com*

DR. JOHN DOUILLARD'S LIFESPA
PROGRAMS AND SERVICES

Education
LifeSpa School of Ayurveda — Ayurvedic Massage certification
Body, Mind, and Sport Personal Trainer certification
The 3–Season Diet weight loss programs
LifeSpa's Ayurvedic online training programs for healthcare
    professionals — free with wholesale accounts

Educational Materials
The 3–Season Diet: Eat the way nature intended
Body, Mind, and Sport: The mind-body guide to lifelong health,
    fitness, and your personal best
Invincible Athletics: This audio series is similar to the book *Body,*
    Mind, and Sport with more emphasis on Ayurveda.
The Ayurvedic Pulse Reading Course: This course will take you step by
    step into an understanding of Ayurveda and pulse diagnosis

Products
Complete Ayurvedic herbal line
Preservative-free skin care products
Books and tapes by Dr. Douillard

Services
Panchakarma
Dayspa treatments
Chiropractic
Ayurvedic consultations
Telephone consultations

www.LifeSpa.com

Convenient online ordering

Medicine Chest: Determine which herbs are best for your condition and take an active role in your own healing. Descriptions, links to articles, recommended dosages, and precautions.

Library: Find articles written by Dr. John Douillard on subjects such as diet, health conditions, herbs, and more.